ANALYTICAL TECHNIQUES IN
ANIMAL NUTRITION RESEARCH

ANALYTICAL TECHNIQUES IN ANIMAL NUTRITION RESEARCH

T.M. Prabhu *M.V.Sc., Ph.D.*
Associate Professor and Head
Department of Animal Nutrition, Veterinary College,
KVAFSU, Hassan-573 201, Karnataka (India)

K.Chandrapal Singh *M.V.Sc., MS (Canada), Ph.D.*
Professor and Head
Department of Animal Nutrition, Veterinary College,
KVAFSU, Bengaluru-560 024, Karnataka (India)

New India Publishing Agency
Pitam Pura, New Delhi-110 088

Published by
Sumit Pal Jain *for*

New India Publishing Agency

101, Vikas Surya Plaza, CU Block, L.S.C. Mkt.,
Pitam Pura, New Delhi 110 088, (India)
Ph.: 011-27341616, Fax: 011-27341717, Mob.: 09717133558
Email: info@nipabooks.com
Web: www.nipabooks.com

© Authors, **2013**

All rights reserved, no part of this publication may be reproduced, stored in a retrieval system or transmitted in any form or by any means, electronic, mechanical, photocopying, recording or otherwise without the prior written permission of the publisher/editor.

This book contains information obtained from authentic and highly regarded sources. Reasonable efforts have been made to publish reliable data and information, but the authors / editor(s) / contributors and publisher cannot assume responsibility for the validity of all materials or the consequences of their use. The authors / editor(s) / contributors and publisher have attempted to trace and acknowledge the copyright holders of all material reproduced in this publication and apologize to copyright holders if permission and acknowledgements to publish in this form have not been given. If any copyright material has not been acknowledged please write and let us know so we may rectify it.

ISBN : 978-93-81450-50-5

Typeset at: Elegant Printographics # 98 91 24 73 05
Printed at: Jai Bharat Printing Press, Delhi

Karnataka Veterinary, Animal & Fisheries Sciences University
P. B. No. 6, Nandinagar, Bidar - 585 401, Karnataka

Prof. Suresh S. Honnappagol
Ph.D., PGDAR, PHAVSC, PGACP, FIAAVR
Vice Chancellor

Ph: 08482 245264
Fax: 08482 245107
e-mail: vckvafsy@yahoo.co.in
sskvafsu@yahoo.co.in
www.kvafsu.edu.in

No. VC/LM-VCH/2012-13 | II - 2863
Ref.:

Date: 28th June, 2012

Foreword

I am very happy to go through the Laboratory Manual on "Analytical Techniques in Animal Nutrition Research" prepared by Dr. Prabhu, T.M., Assocaite Professor & Head, Dept. Animal Nutrition, Veterinary College, KVAFSU, Hassan and Dr. Chandrapal Singh, K., Professor & Head, Dept. Animal Nutrition, Veterinary College, KVAFSU, Bengaluru, Karnataka. The topics covered in the manual ranged from commonly used routine analytical procedures in Animal Nutrition laboratories to the latest techniques required for specialized studies with ruminants.

The rich experience in teaching and research facilitated the faculty to prepare the topics for easy adaptation by post-graduate scholars of Animal Nutrition and other related disciplines from Veterinary / Agricultural Universities and Research Institutes of India and other developing countries. This may also be helpful for use by the feed compounding industries.

It is my immense pleasure to recommend this laboratory manual for day-to-day use by scholars, teachers and research workers in the field of Animal Nutrition and related disciplines.

(Suresh S. Honnappagol)
Vice Chancellor
Karnataka Veterinary,
Animal and Fisheries Sciences
University, BIDAR

PREFACE

The livestock industry is growing in a much accelerated rate to meet the increased quality protein demand of our ever increasing population. The cost of feeding the animals and birds comes to nearly 70-75% of the total production cost of animal produce. Hence, assessing the quality of raw materials and judicious use of these ingredients in the preparation of an economical and balanced feed is very important. Further, the quality of raw materials show wide variation in the nutrient content. In such a situation precise measurement of the nutrient content is not only an important factor but the time involvement is also very important.

In this manual efforts have been made to cover a wide range of topics including detergent system of feed analysis, *in vitro, in situ* and *in vivo* studies to evaluate feedstuffs for their nutritive worth. Analysis of rumen liquor for fraction of VFA's enzymatic activity of various metabolites and estimation of rumen fluid volume and its flow rate are covered in depth. It was followed by estimation of anti-nutritional / toxic factors in various un-conventional feeds using HPLC / Spectrophotometer, detail analysis of milk and body condition scoring for dairy cattle are included as assessment of these parameters are important in Ruminant Nutrition Research.

Laboratory techniques are subject to continuous modification and improvement and this collection will be no exception. All the methods which are described, have been in regular use and therefore may be relied upon to obtain positive results. Although, necessary practical work is included, the exhaustive details have been avoided, since the manual is primarily meant for postgraduate scholars, teachers, scientists and feed industry personnel use. It is possible that in spite of our best efforts this compilation has still some shortcomings and mistakes / faults. We respectfully look to our generous readers, fellow teachers and scientists to point to us any fault or omission that may have crept inadvertently.

An attempt has been made to incorporate into this manual a variety of important source materials that ordinarily can be found in many different locations. There is no claim made for originality in the essential and basic subject matter, but approach to the demonstration and performing of various research methodologies, its manner of treatment and presentation is entirely based on our own experiences.

We wish to place on record our indebtedness to Prof. Suresh, S. Honnappagol, the Vice-Chancellor, Dr. S. Yathiraj, Dr. M.S. Vasanth, Dean and Dr. U. Krishnamoorthy, Head, Division of Animal Science, KVAFSU, Bidar for their encouragement. The assistance and support of the publisher is most gratefully acknowledged.

2012

Prabhu, T.M.
Chandrapal Singh, K.

CONTENTS

Foreword		v
Preface		vii
1	CHEMICAL ANALYSIS	1
2	*IN VITRO* RUMEN STUDIES	13
3	*IN SITU* DACRON BAG STUDIES	23
4	NITROGEN FRACTIONATION BY CHEMICAL AND *IN VITRO* METHODS	35
5	ENZYMATIC METHODS	39
6	HOHENHEIM GAS TEST - OTHER APPLICATIONS	43
7	RUMEN LIQUOR ANALYSIS	49
8	ESTIMATION OF RUMEN MICROBIAL PROTEIN PRODUCTION FROM PURINE DERIVATIVES IN URINE	77
9	RUMEN FLUID VOLUME & ITS FLOW RATE	85
10	CHROMATOGRAPHIC TECHNIQUES AND ITS APPLICATION IN ANIMAL NUTRITION RESEARCH	87
11	FRACTIONATION OF VOLATILE FATTY ACIDS WITH GAS LIQUID CHROMATOGRAPHY	95
12	HIGH PERFORMANCE LIQUID CHROMATOGRAPHIC ANALYSIS OF KARANJIN IN KARANJ (HONGE) SEED CAKE	101

13	ESTIMATION OF AZADIRACHTIN IN NEEM SEED CAKE BY HPLC	103
14	ESTIMATION OF RICIN IN CASTOR BEAN MEAL BY SDS-PAGE	107
15	UV VISIBLE SPECTROPHOTOMETRIC METHOD OF ESTIMATION OF GOSSYPOL	111
16	ATOMIC ABSORPTION SPECTROPHOTOMETRY: APPLICATION IN ANIMAL NUTRITION RESEARCH	117
17	NEAR INFRA RED SPECTROSCOPY (NIRS) : APPLICATION IN ANIMAL NUTRITION RESEARCH	123
18	ESTIMATION OF ANTINUTRITIONAL FACTORS IN FEEDS & FODDERS	131
19	METHOD OF CONDUCTING DIGESTION/ METABOLISM (BALANCE) TRIAL ON EXPERIMENTAL ANIMALS	157
20	MISCELLANEOUS	163
21	ANALYSIS OF MILK	167
22	BODY CONDITION SCORING FOR DAIRY CATTLE	173
23	SOME EQUIVALENTS AND FORMULAE FREQUENTLY USED IN RUMINANT FEED EVALUATION	175
	GENERAL INSTRUCTIONS	177
	REFERENCES	179

Chapter 1

CHEMICAL ANALYSIS

The chemical composition and digestibility of feedstuffs influence their nutritive value for animal production. Therefore, assessment of nutritive value of feedstuffs continues to be one of the top priority areas in animal production research. Although traditionally the feedstuffs were evaluated by performance studies and digestion trials, such techniques are expensive and requires more time and labour. Continued search for alternatives to animal feeding experiments have led to the development of feed evaluation systems that are rapid and economical.

In general, there are two kinds of laboratory analyses — Chemical analyses and Biological tests with rumen micro-organisms or purified enzymes. Biological tests give direct estimates of digestibility, but are lengthier and more expensive. Chemical analyses are cheaper and rapid, but do not give direct estimates of nutritive value. The statistical association between the chemical components and quality need to be established to predict the nutritive value.

1.1 Proximate Analysis

This is the conventional system that has been in use for more than 140 years. In this system, the feed components are classified into six groups called proximate principles. They are water, ether extract, crude fibre, crude protein, total ash and nitrogen free extractives (NFE). It consists of the following steps:

A. Determination of water by drying at 100°C and obtaining dry residue,
B. Ether extraction of the dry residue for estimation of lipids,

C. Reflux of fat-extracted residue for 30 minute with 1.25% sulphuric acid followed by 30 minute with 1.25% sodium hydroxide. The insoluble residue is dried, weighed and ashed and the incinerated organic matter reported as crude fibre,
D. Determination of crude protein (nitrogen in feed x 6.25) and
E. Incinerated (550°C for 3 hours) residue of feed expressed as total ash, and,
F. The calculation of NFE as the dry matter not accounted for by the sum of ether extract, crude fibre, ash and crude protein.

Much of the data available on feed composition are based on proximate analysis. Although this system is simple,. it only gives information on chemical composition but not on digestibility. Besides, the system has other drawbacks with a potential for misinterpretation of nutritive value (Van Soest, 1994). The detailed procedures for the analysis of proximate principles are described in a separate manual.

1.2 Detergent System of Feed Analysis

This system was developed in an attempt to group feed components on the basis of their digestibility, and to find a replacement for the carbohydrate fractionation into crude fibre and nitrogen free extractives in the proximate analysis. This system attempts to classify feed dry matter according to their uniformity in digestibility (Table 1.2.1). The basic scheme of forage analysis by detergent system is presented in (Table 1.2.2).

Neutral Detergent Fibre : Extraction of feed with a neutral (pH 7.0) solution of sodium lauryl sulphate and ethylenediamine tetraacetic acid will recover major cell wall components such as lignin, cellulose and hemicellulose. The minor cell wall components such as protein, lignin bound nitrogen, minerals and cuticle are also recovered. However, pectin which is a cell wall component is not recovered.

Common contaminants of the neutral detergent residue include starch, animal keratin and soil minerals. The interference of starch can be eliminated through pre-treatment or concomitant treatment with amylases. The presence of keratins in feedstuffs is rare unless animal products are incorporated in mixed feeds. In faeces, hair and epithelial sloughings contribute to keratin. The interference of keratins can be eliminated with the use of sodium sulphite. However, since sulphite also solubilises lignin, the use of sulphite is not recommended, if the cell wall preparation is to be used for further analysis of other components.

Chemical Analysis

Table 1.2.1 : Division of feed organic matter by detergent system

Fraction	Components	Availabilty
Cell contents (Soluble in neutral detergent)	Lipids, Sugars, organic aids and water soluble matter, Pectin, Starch, Non-protein, Soluble protein	Almost completely digestible-not lignified
Cell wall constituents (fibre insoluble in neutral detergent)		Partially digestible according to the degree of lignification
1. Soluble in acid detergent	Hemicellulose, Fibre bound proteins	
2. Acid-detergent fibre	Cellulose, lignin, lignified nitrogen	

Van Soest, 1982

Table 1.2.2 : Basic scheme of forage analysis using detergents

Fraction	Reagents	Treatment	Yeild
Neutral-Detergent Fibre (NDF)	Na lauryl sulphate, EDTA, pH 7.0	Boil 1 h.	Plant cell wall less pectins
Acid-Detergent Fibre (ADF)	Cetyl trimethyl-ammonium bromide in 1N H_2SO_4	Boil 1 h	Lignocellulose + insoluble material
Unavailable nitrogen	Acid detergent	Kjeldahl N determination on ADF	Maillard products and lignified N
Lignin	72% H_2SO_4	3 h, 20°C	Crude lignin
Cellulose	None	Ash residue from ligning step	Loss in weight
Silica (SiO_2)	Conc. HBr (48%)	Treat ash drop wish 1 h, 25°C	Residue in SiO_2
Hemicellulose	None	Calculate as NDF-ADF	

Van Soest, 1982

The natural mineral components of the cell wall are recovered in the neutral detergent residue. Much of the biogenic silica is solubilised in neutral detergent extraction. The contaminant soil silica is insoluble. Therefore the neutral detergent residual silica is an estimate of soil contamination of sample.

Acid Detergent Fibre : Feed components of variable digestibility and completely indigestible components are recovered in acid detergent extraction. The acid detergent (cetyl trimethyl ammonium bromide in 1 N H_2SO_4) divides these into soluble and insoluble fractions. Acid soluble fractions include hemicelluloses and cell wall proteins, whereas the insoluble fraction includes the cellulose and least digestible non-carbohydrate fractions. Extraction of feedstuffs with acid detergent solution has the advantage of removing substances that interfere with the estimation of refractory components so that ADF residue is useful for the sequential estimations of lignin, cutin, cellulose, indigestible nitrogen and silica. Silica is almost completely recovered in acid detergent residue.

Interferences in Estimating Hemicellulose by Difference Between NDF and ADF : Neutral detergent dissolves pectin, much of silica and tannins whereas acid detergent precipitates silica, tannin-protein complexes and to some extent pectins. Acid detergent residues are usually lower in protein than neutral detergent residues. Therefore, the presence of pectin, tannin and silica influence the hemicellulose values calculated by the difference between NDF and ADF (Table 1.2.3.).

Table 1.2.3 : Interferences in the estimation of hemicellulose as the difference between NDF and ADF

Fraction	Recovery in		Effect on estimate
	NDF	ADF	
Cell wall proteins	Recovered	Largely recovered	Increase
Biogenic silica	Considerable recovery	Quantitative recovery	Decrease
Pectin	Dissolved	Partial precipitation	Decrease
Tannin	Precipitation as protein complex	Partly dissolved	Increase

Van Soest, 1994

Procedure for determination of fibre fractions and their application in feed evaluation (Goering and Van Soest, 1970)

Reagents

1. Neutral detergent solution

Distilled water	L	1
Sodium lauryl sulphate	g	30.00
Disodium ethylene diamine teteraacetate (EDTA dehydrate crystals)	g	18.61
Sodium borate decahydrate, reagent grade	g	6.81
Disodium hydrogen phosphate, anhydrous reagent grade	g	4.56
2-ethoxyethanol (ethylene glycol monoethyl ether) purified grade	ml	10.00

Chemical Analysis

Put EDTA and $Na_2B_4O7.10H_2O$ together in a large beaker, add some of the distilled water, and heat until dissolved, then add to solution containing sodium lauryl sulphate and 2-ethoxyethanol (ethylene glycol monoethyl ether). Put Na_2HPO_4 in beaker, add some of the distilled water, and heat until dissolved; then add to solution containing other ingredients. Check pH to range 6.9 to 7.01. If solution is properly made, pH adjustment will rarely be required.

2. Acetone

Use grade that is free from colour and leaves no residue upon evaporation.

3. Acid detergent solution

Acid detergent solution	L	1
Sulphuric acid, reagent grade (100 = per cent assay)	g	49.04
Cetyl trimethyl ammonium bromide (CTAB technical grade)	g	20.00

Weigh sulphuric acid and make up volume with distilled water at 20°C. Check normality by titration before addition of detergent. Then add CTAB and stir.

4. Sulphuric acid 72 per cent by weight — calculate grams acid and water needed in 1 L of solution by:

$$\frac{100 \times 98.08 \times 12 \text{ moles}}{H_2SO_4 \text{ assay (per cent)}} = \text{grams acid needed}$$

$(1{,}000 \times 1.634)^*$ - grams acid = grams water needed
* Weight of 1 litre of 72 per cent H_2SO_4

Weigh amount of water into a 1 L MCA volumetric flask (with a bulb in the neck) and add the calculated amount of H_2SO_4 slowly with occasional swirling. Caution ! Flaks must be cooled in a water bath in order to add the required weight of sulphuric acid. Cool to 20°C and check if the volume is correct. If the volume is too small, take out about 1.5 ml and add 2.5 ml water. Repeat if necessary. If the volume is too large, take out 5 ml and add 4.45 ml H_2SO_4. Meniscus should be within a 0.5 cm of calibration mark at 20°C.

5. Saturated potassium permanganate

Distilled water	L	1
$KMnO_4$ reagent grade	g	50.0
Ag_2SO_4 reagent grade g	g	0.05

Dissolve $KMnO_4$ and Ag_2SO_4 in distilled water in distilled water. Keep out of direct sunlight. Add silver sulphate to dehalogenate the reagent.

6. Lignin buffer solution (1 L)

Ferric nitrate nonahydrate	g	6.00
Silver nitrate	g	0.15
Acetic acid, glacial	ml	500
Potassium acetate	g	5.00
Tertiary bytyl alcohol	ml	400
Distilled water	ml	100

Dissolve ferric nitrate nonahydrate [$(FeNO_3)_3$ $9H_2O$] and silver nitrate in distilled water. Combine with acetic acid and potassium acetate. Add tertiary butyl alcohol and mix. Use grade of acid and solvent passing dichromate test (ACS).

7. Combined Permanganate Solution

Combine and mix saturated potassium permanganate and lignin buffer solution in the ratio of 2:1, by volume, before use. Unused mixed solution may be kept about a week in a refrigerator in the absence of light. Solution is usable if purple and contain no precipitate. Old solution assume a reddish colour and should be discarded.

8. Demineralising solution (1 L)

Oxalic acid dehydrate	g	50.0
95 per cent ethanol	ml	750
Concentrated (about 12N) hydrochloric acid	ml	50
Distilled water	ml	250

Dissolve oxalic acid dehydrate in 95 per cent ethanol. Add concentrated hydrochloric acid and distilled water and mix.

9. Ethanol 80 per cent (1 L)

95 per cent ethanol	ml	845
Distilled water	ml	155

10. Hydrobromic acid reagent grade

11. Cleaning solution

Distilled water	L	1
Disodium ethylene, diamine tetraacetate (EDTA) dehydrate crystal	g	5
Trisodium phosphate, laboratory grade	g	50
Potassium hydroxide	g	200

Procedures

Neutral Detergent Fibre (Cell Wall)

Reagents required 1 and 2

1. Weigh 0.5 to 1.0 g air dry sample ground to pass 20 to 30 mesh (1mm) or equivalent into a beaker of the refluxing apparatus.
2. Add in order, 100 ml cold (room temperature) neutral detergent solution, heat to boiling in 5 to 10 minutes. Reduce heat as boiling begins, to avoid foaming. Adjust boiling to an even level and reflux for 60 minutes, timed from onset of boiling.
3. Place previously tared Gooch crucibles (Grade 2) on filter manifold. Swirl beaker to suspend solids, and fill crucible. Do not admit vacuum until after crucible has been filled. Use low vacuum at first and increase it only as more force is needed. Rinse sample into crucible with minimum of hot (90°C to 100°C) water. Remove vacuum, break up mat, and fill crucible with hot water. Filter liquid and repeat washing procedure.
4. Wash twice with acetone in same manner and suck dry. Dry crucibles at 100°C for 8 hours or overnight and weigh.
5. Report yield of recovered neutral detergent fibre as per cent of dry matter. Estimate cell solubles by subtracting this value from 100.
6. Ash residue in the crucible for 3 hours at 500°C to 550°C and weigh. Report ash content as ash in neutral detergent.

Acid Detergent Fibre

Reagents required: 2 and 3

1. Weigh 1 g air dry sample ground to pass 20 to 30 mesh (1 mm) screen or the approximate equivalent of wet material into a beaker suitable for refluxing.
2. Add 100 ml cold (room temperature) acid detergent solution. Heat to boiling in 5 to 10 minutes. Reduce heat as boiling begins, to avoid foaming. Reflux 60 minutes from onset of boiling; adjust boiling to a slow, even level.
3. Follow steps 3 and 4 of NDF determination. Recovered fibre is ADF.

Acid Detergent Lignin

Reagents required; 2, 3, and 4

In the acid detergent lignin procedure, the acid detergent fibre (ADF) procedure is used as a preparatory step. The detergent removes the protein and other acid-soluble material that would interfere with the lignin determination. The ADF residue consists of cellulose, lignin, cutin and acid insoluble ash (mainly silica). Treatment with 72 per cent sulphuric acid dissolves cellulose. Ashing of the residue will determine the crude lignin including cutin. For silica determination and separation of cutin and lignin, see the permanganate and acid detergent cutin procedures.

1. Prepare The Acid Detergent Fibre.
2. Cover the contents of the crucible with cooled (15°C) 72 per cent H_2SO_4 and stir with a glass rod to a smooth paste, breaking all lumps. Fill crucible about half full with acid and stir. Let glass rod remain in crucible; refill with 72 per cent H_2SO_4 and stir at hourly intervals as acid drains away. Crucibles do not need to be kept full at all the times. Three additions suffice. Keep crucible at 20°C to 23°C. After 3 hours, filter off as much acid as possible with vacuum; then wash contents with hot water until free from acid. Rinse and remove stirring rod.
3. Dry crucible at 100°C and weigh.
4. Ignite crucible in a muffle furnace at 500°C to 550°C for 3 hours and then cool to 100°C and weigh. Loss on ignition represents lignin.

Permanganate Lignin, Cellulose, Insoluble Ash and Silica

Reagents required: 2, 3, 5 through 10.

1. Dry samples at less than 65°C and grind through 20 to 30 mesh (1 mm) screen, Prepare and determine acid detergent fibre according to standard procedure. Use 1 g of sample, except on samples containing a high amount of lignin (15% or more) use 0.5 g sample. Place previously weighed crucibles in a shallow enamel pan containing cold water to a depth of about 1 cm. Fibre in crucibles should not be wet.
2. Add about 25 ml of combined saturated potassium permanganate and lignin buffer solution (2:1 by volume) to the crucibles in the enamel pan containing cold water. Adjust level (2-3 cm) of water in pan to reduce flow of solution out of crucibles. Place a short glass rod in each crucible to stir contents, to break lumps and to draw permanganate solution upon sides of crucibles to wet all particles.
3. Allow crucibles to stand at 20°C to 25°C for 90±10 minutes; add more mixed permanganate solution if necessary. Purple colour must be present all the times.
4. Remove crucibles to filtering apparatus. Suck dry. Do not wash. Place in a clean enamel pan, and fill crucibles not more than half full with demineralising solution. Demineralising solution may be added directly to crucibles in case filtering is difficult. Care must be taken to avoid spillage by foaming. After about 5 minutes, suck dry on filter and refill half full with demineralising solution. Repeat after second interval if solution is very brown. Rinse sides of crucibles with solution from a wash bottle with a fine stream. Treat until fibre is white. Total time required is about 20 to 30 minutes.
5. Fill and thoroughly wash crucible and contents with 80 per cent ethanol. Suck dry and repeat two times. Wash twice in similar manner with acetone. Suck dry.
6. Dry at 100°C overnight and weigh. Calculate lignin content as loss in weight from acid detergent fibre.
7. Ash at 500°C for 3 hours, cool and weigh. Calculate residual ash as the difference between this weight and original tare of the crucible. Calculate cellulose by weight loss upon ashing.
8. A presumptive analysis for silica may be obtained by hydrobromic acid treatment of the ashed permanganate lignin of ADF residue. This determination has its greatest value when the residual ash is greater than 2 per cent. Ash and weigh, then add enough drops of 48 per cent HBr to moisten all particles. Use no more than 4 ml acid. Allow to stand 1 to 2 hours. Add more drops of HBr if much red colour forms. Suck off excess acid on vacuum and wash once with acetone. Use no

water. Dry and ash briefly at 500°C, Cool and weigh. Report silica as the difference between this weight and the original tare.

Precautions

Crucibles containing fibre of a high lignin content require more permanganate solution; however, avoid additions of more solution than is necessary. Appearance of a yellow or brown colour indicates exhaustion of permanganate. If crucible is full, filter solution off on a vacuum and add more . reagent. A yellow colour persisting after treatment of fibre with demineralising solution indicates incomplete removal of the lignin. This occurs only in materials of a very high lignin content. Cutin material present in seed coats and other plant parts is not oxidised by permanganate; thus it is neither determined as lignin nor bleached with the treatments. Seed coats appear as coloured flecks among white cellulose particles, and thus they should not be confused with incomplete oxidation.

Excessive flow of permanganate solution through the crucibles should be avoided with samples of low lignin content, particularly in samples of immature grasses. With these, a single addition of permanganate solution suffices. Fibre from immature grasses is very rapidly delignified, and therefore, there is danger of loss of cellulosic carbohydrates if the flow is too great. Reduction in flow is accomplished by adjusting the water level in the pan to near that in crucibles. These precautions are not needed with the demineralising solution.

Acid Detergent Cutin

Reagents required: 2 through 10.

The fraction of plant material referred to as cutin is the fraction that is not oxidised by $KMnO_4$ and resists hydrolysis by 72 per cent H_2SO_4. This fraction can be very large, as in some seed hulls, or nor important, as in the common forages. The relation of cutin to the nutritive value of other plant constituents is not understood. However cutin factor is resistant to microbial degradation.

1. Follow procedure for $KMnO_4$, lignin and cellulose preparation up to the step where lignin can be calculated but the residue has not been ashed (steps 1— 6).
2. Treat the unashed residue with 72 per cent H_2SO_4 as in the acid detergent lignin procedure.
3. Calculate lignin as loss in weight upon ashing.

Chemical Analysis

Crucible Cleaning

Reagents required: 11
1. Empty contents and ash crucibles briefly, 1 to 2 hours, at 500°C to 550°C (not necessary if crucible is already ashed in lignin or silica determination).
2. Wash crucible with tap water.
3. Force distilled water upward through the crucible; use a No. 7 rubber stopper with tube through middle connected to the distilled water outlet. Rinse outside with distilled water and place in oven. Proceed to next step if the crucible does not give normal filtering properties.
4. Place crucible that has been ashed in 500°C to 550°C in a shallow enamel pan,. Add about 50 ml crucible cleaning solution to each crucible. Heat (such as steam bath) should be placed under the pan. Let cleaning solution filter through the crucible. Bore hole in a No. 9½ rubber stopper and insert one end of a 50 ml pipette and attach a tube to the upper end of the pipette. Place the stopper assembly in the top of the crucible and apply vacuum until the crucible is approximately one-half full of cleaning solution. Wait for solution to filter through the crucible again. Refill the crucible with the solution again. The cleaning solution may be saved and reused.
5. Repeat steps 2 and 3.

Acid Detergent Insoluble Nitrogen

Reagents required: 2 and 3.

Heat-drying of forages at temperatures above 50°C shows analytically significant increases in yield of lignin and fibre. The increased yield of acid detergent fibre (ADF) can be accounted for largely by the production of artefact lignin via the nonenzymatic browning reaction. Value for ADF and lignin in dried forages can be corrected on the basis of the nitrogen content of the ADF. The nitrogen content of the ADF is suggested as a sensitive assay for non-enzymatic browning due to overheating of the feeds.

1. Follow step 1 and 2 of acid detergent fibre procedure using a 2 g sample.
2. Filter with suction on previously tared 12.5 cm Whatman No. 54 paper. Fold paper into a cone and use 60° angle funnel and a filter cone (Fisher No. 9-760) to protect tip.
3. Wash paper with hot water and then with acetone until acid free. Dry at 100°C for 8 hours or overnight and weigh.
4. Transfer paper residue into kjeldahl flask. Run nitrogen on residue according to standard kjeldahl procedure

1.3. Prediction of energy content by summative equations of detergent system (SEDS).

The ME in roughages and compound feeds can be estimated using different summative equations (Van Soest, 1971; Van Soest 1994; Conrad et al., 1984; Girard and Dupuis, 1988; Giger-Riverdin et al., 1994)

Roughages (Goering and Van Soest, 1970; Van Soest, 1971).

TDDM = (NDS x 0.98)+(NDF x ((147.3 — (78.9 Log_{10} ((L+BS)x 100/ADF)))/100)) - (SSx1.4) (i)
ADDM = TDDM — (365.7-0.275TDDM) (ii)
TDN = ADDM — (TA-TS) + 1.25 EE + 19 (iii)

Compound Feeds (Giger-Reverdin *et al.*, 1994)

ME = 13.38 + 0.0118 EE - .00547NDF + .0065ADF - .0378ADL + .00291CP (iv)

Where, ME = Metabolisable energy (MJ Kg^{-1} DM), TDDM, ADDM, TDN, EE, NDS, NDF, BS, ADL, ADF, SS, TS, TA, CP are true digestible dry matter, apparent digestible dry matter, total digestible nutrient, ether extract, neutral detergent solubles, neutral detergent fibre, biogenic silica, acid detergent lignin, acid detergent fibre, sand silica, total silica, total ash and crude protein respectively, in g Kg^{-1} DM.

Note : NDF ash = Sand silica, ADF ash = Total silica, ADF ash — NDF ash = Biogenic silica

Data set to demonstrate calculations:

Table 1.2.4: Chemical composition (g, $Kg^{-1}DM$) and Metabolisable Energy (ME, MJ, $Kg^{-1}DM$) predicted from SEDS for roughage and compounded feed mixture

Constituent	Finger millet straw	Compounded feed mixture
Neutral detergent fibre	764	368
Acid detergent fibre	475	243
Acid detergent lignin	59	82
Total ash	72	109
Sand Silica	15	12
Biogenic silica	5	17
Ether extract	13	27
Crude protein	51	196
ME(SEDS)	6.18	10.7

Chapter 2

IN VITRO RUMEN STUDIES

The estimation of digestibility by feeding trials with sheep or other ruminants is laborious and requires large quantities of feed. Therefore, the chemical composition of feedstuffs are used to predict digestibility by making use of established mathematical relationship between digestibility and composition. However, since the relationship between digestibility and chemical composition varies with the type of feedstuffs, for each group of feedstuffs, mathematical equations will have to be developed by relating chemical composition with *in vivo* digestibility. In spite of this, the errors associated with this approach of predicting digestibility is large. This has led to the development of techniques that would mimic digestive function of the ruminant in the laboratory.

In vitro methods of feed evaluation using rumen fluid and/or digestive enzymes are the most widely used techniques in ruminant feed evaluation. Although, the technique adopted in different laboratories differ, the principle of the technique is essentially a partially simulated rumen environment *in vitro* by incubating rumen fluid anaerobically in buffered medium at 39°C for variable period of time. Currently the most commonly used rumen *in vitro* techniques are,
(a) Two stage digestion (Tilley and Terry, 1963)
(b) Modified two stage digestion (Goering and Van Soest, 1970)
(c) Hohenheim gas test (Menke et al., 1979)

2.1 *In vitro* Two Stage Digestion (Tilley and Terry, 1963)

This technique attempts to simulate rumen digestion followed by gastric digestion. A known quantity of feed sample is incubated with rumen inoculum at 39°C under carbon dioxide for 48 hours followed by acidification with HCl, and incubation with pepsin enzyme at 39°C for 48 hours. The undigested feed residue is recovered either by filtration through previously tared Whatman No. 4, 41, or 54 filter paper or by centrifugation at 15000 x g for 30 minutes, with parallel running of incubations without feed samples to serve as blank. The feed component not recovered is regarded as digestible dry matter.

In the first stage of rumen digestion, feed is subjected to microbial digestion resulting in microbial cell synthesis and metabolic wastes such as volatile fatty acids and gases. In the second stage, the unfermented feed components and the microbial cells are digested by the pepsin HCl acid. Therefore, the undigested residue from these incubations are comparable to the faecal component of this feed (except for endogenous matter), if a digestion trial is carried out *in vivo*. Thus, the digestibility estimates obtained by this technique is comparable to apparent digestibility. Therefore, this technique gives digestibility of feed highly correlated with *in vivo* values, with numerically small difference between the two values. Digestibilities by Tilley and Terry technique may average about two points higher than the *in vivo* apparent digestibility values. This is within the standard deviation of most *in vivo* digestion trials and in fact most people using the *in vitro* method apply no statistical correction.

2.2 Modified *In vitro* Two Stage Digestion Technique (Goering and Van Soest, 1970)

The total duration of incubation in *in vitro* two stage digestion technique (Tilley and Terry, 1963) .lasts for 96 hours. In the modified *in vitro* two stage digestion technique, the acid pepsin digestion of 48 hours is replaced by neutral detergent (ND) extraction. Following the first stage of digestion with rumen inoculum for 48 hours, the contents of the incubation is subjected to extraction in ND solution to recover ND insoluble residue. While pepsin HCl digestion solubilises potential digestible components of feed and all of microbial matter including indigestible microbial cell walls. Therefore, the undigested residue obtained after ND extraction, is completely of feed origin and represents true indigestible component. Thus the digestibility obtained by this technique is true digestibility and these values are comparable to *in vivo* true digestibility. Since, the conventionally used index of feed quality is the apparent digestibility, true digestibility estimates are converted into apparent digestibility by subtraction of a metabolic value of 12.9.

Procedure (Tilley and Terry, 1963; Goering and Van Soest, 1970)

Materials

1. Rumen-content source from an animal on a high cell-wall roughage (preferably a rumen cannulated animal)
2. Erlenmeyer flasks, 125 ml (pyrex, requiring No.6 stoppers).
3. Shaking water bath at 40°C with holder for 18 flasks.
4. Manifold for 18 flasks constructed over water bath.
5. Waring blender
6. CO_2 source.
7. Cheese cloth.
8. Glass wool and enclosed funnel assemble.
9. Automatic syringe, 10 ml.
10. Glassware refluxing apparatus as used for detergent preparations.

Description

Fermentations are conducted in 125 ml. Pyrex Erlenmeyer flasks (wide-mouth); 0.5 g substrate, 40 ml medium, and 10 ml inoculum are used. Fermentation flasks are placed in shaking water bath (capacity 18) and closed with No. 6 rubber stoppers. Stoppers are fitted with three openings; an inlet tube, a Bunsen valve-both flush with the bottom of the stopper-and a gassing tube connected to a common manifold. The inlet tube is closed on the outside with a rubber sleeve and glass rod. The gassing tube should stop about 1 cm above the surface of the liquid. The manifold is connected to a supply of carbon dioxide and in parallel with a water manometer with a capacity of 60 cm water pressure.

Reagents
- Trypticase-A pancreatic digest of casein, USP
- Sodium sulphide nonahydrate-Reagent grade
- 1 N Sodium hydroxide — Dissolve 4 g in water and dilute to a litre.
- Cysteine — HCl
- Resazurin-0.1 per cent w/v solution
- 6 N HCl—Dilute concentrated HCl (about 12 N) with an equal amount of water. Need not be standardised.
- Pepsin-NF (Fisher Scientific)
- Toluene- Commercial grade.

In vitro Rumen Buffer Solution

Distilled water	L	1
Ammonium bicarbonate	g	4
Sodium bicarbonate	g	35

In vitro Rumen Macromineral Solution

Distilled water	L	1
Na_2HPO_4	g	5.7
KH_2PO_4 anhydrous	g	6.2
$MgSO_4\,7H_2O$	g	0.6

In vitro Micromineral Solution

$CaCl_2.2H_2O$	g	13.2
$MnCl_2.4H_2O$	g	10.0
$CoCl_2.6H_2O$	g	1.0
$FeCl_3.6H_2O$	g	8.0

Add to volumetric flask and bring volume to 100 ml with distilled water.

Incubation

The first five steps are common for both procedures.
1. Weigh 0.5 g sample (20 mesh or 1 mm) into 125 ml Erlenmeyer flask.
2. Prepare medium - Add in order trypticase, 400 ml water and 0.1 ml micromineral solution, and agitate to dissolve. Then add 200 ml buffer solution, 200 ml macromineral solution, and 1 ml resazurin. Mix and add 40 ml per 125 ml flask.
3. Equilibration - Assemble and put stoppers and flasks in bath, admit carbon dioxide (about 30 to 40 cm water) and check Bunsen valves. Open the inlet tubes and swirl flask while open and then close. Next prepare the reducing solution. Add 625 mg cysteine hydrochloric acid, 95 ml water, 4 ml 1N sodium hydroxide and dissolve; then add 625 mg sodium sulphide nonahydrate and dissolve. Reduce carbon dioxide pressure to 3 or 4 cm, and inject 2 ml reducing solution through the inlet tube with an automatic syringe; open and close each tube in turn. Swirl all flasks. Watch for reduction of medium, which is a change from a red colour (oxidised) to colourless (reduced).
4. Prepare inoculum — Collect ingesta from a fistulated animal in a litre beaker, fill, cover with a watch glass to eliminate air space. Discard the top layer of the ingesta. And blend 400 ml of the remainder in a waring blender for 2 minutes under carbon dioxide. Squeeze the blended mass through cheese cloth and filter through glass wool into a warm flask; thereafter keep the filtrate under carbon dioxide. Inoculate 10 ml of the filtrate with an automatic syringe through inlet tubes of each fermentation flask.

In-Vitro Rumen Studies

5. Fermentation — Seal tubes and incubate 48 hours with shaking at a rate not to produce splashing. Adjust carbon dioxide pressure to 2 cm water. At the end of fermentation one of the procedures, step 6 or step 7 can be followed. (step 6 - Tilley and Terry (1963) filtration procedure or step -7 treatment with neutral detergent). Flasks may be stored before proceeding with step 6 or 7. Add 1 ml toluene as a preservative and refrigerate. Stopper with cork.
6. Tilley and terry procedure — Add 2 ml 6 N HCl to each flask carefully to avoid excessive farming. (This is sufficient to lower pH below 2) Add 0.5 g pepsin (may be measured with a scoop). Swirl to dissolve. Add 1 ml toluene, replace flask in a water bath, and incubate 48 hours. Remove flasks from water bath and filter on previously tared Whatman No. 4, 41 or 54 filter paper without suction. Rinse filter twice by filling (almost to overflowing) and allowing to drain and air dry. Fold paper, dry at 100°C and weigh. Dry matter on paper is done on separate circles. Use dry matter factor to calculate dry weight for tared paper circles used in filtering. Separate blanks containing inoculum and medium only, must be run simultaneously. Whatman No. 4, 41 or 54 filter paper and a common forage such as orchard grass are used as standards.
7. Neutral detergent procedure for estimation of true digestibility — Remove flasks from water bath after digestion or from refrigerator if stored. Wash with 100 ml neutral detergent solution into 600 ml Berzelius beaker to make a total volume of 150 ml. Add 2 ml decahydronaphthalene. Reflux for 1 hour, and filter on previously tared 50 ml., 40 mm plate, coarse porocity fritted-glass crucibles. Wash twice with hot water and twice with acetone, and suck dry. Dry in oven at 100°C and weigh. Blanks are not necessary.
8. Calculations:
Calculate true dry matter digestibility:
100 — per cent ND residue = true digestibility
Calculate by Tilley and Terry method:
$[1.00-\{(R-F)-blank/oven-drysample weight\}]100 = \%$ digestibility.
Where   R = weight of residue and filter paper
         F = weight of filter paper
Blank value is R — F when substrate is not added to medium.

2.3 Hohenheim Gas Test (Menke et al., 1979; Menke and Steingass, 1988)

In the previously described *in vitro* techniques, the unrecovered substrate in the process of separation of solubles from the insoluble feed components following digestion, is regarded as digestible. This assumption is not necessarily true, because some feed components that are soluble may still remain indigestible and/or interfere in digestion of other components. Therefore, attempts to develop a technique to evaluate feedstuffs based on the ultimate end product of microbial fermentation resulted in the development of Hohenheim Gas Test.

This technique is based on the gas produced (carbon dioxide and methane) during the course of fermentation by the rumen inoculum. Feedstuffs of different digestibilities show marked differences in the rate and amount of gas produced within a stipulated period of time. The gas accumulated in the fermentation vessel originates from the fermentation of the feedstuffs and also from the buffered medium as a consequence of volatile fatty acids displacing the dissolved carbon dioxide (Menke and Steingass, 1988; Blümmel, 1994). Since gas produced is an index of microbial fermentation of feedstuff, cumulative gas production in 24 hours incubation is used as one of the variables to predict apparent digestibility by appropriate regression equation. Therefore, the basic approach in application of gas test to predict apparent digestibility of feedstuffs is similar to that used in the application of chemical analyses to predict digestibility. However, the important difference between the two is that, in gas test, a component of substrate fermented by the microbes is incorporated in prediction equations, which improve the reliability of this technique across a wider variety of feedstuffs.

Procedure (Menke *et al.*, 1979; Menke and Steingass, 1988)

Materials Required

100 ml calibrated syringes, incubator fitted with a rotor or a water bath.

Reagents

1. Micromineral Solution
$CaCl_2.2H_2O$ 13.2 g
$MnCl_2.4H_2O$ 10.0 g
$CoCl_2.6H_2O$ 1.00 g
$FeCl_3.6H_2O$ 8.00 g
Dissolve and make up to 100 ml with distilled water and keep refrigerated.

2. Buffer Solution
$NaHCO_3$ 35 g
NH_4HCO_3 4 g
Dissolve and make up to 1000 ml with distilled water.

3. Macromineral Solution
Na_2HPO_4	5.7 g
KH_2PO_4	6.2 g
$MgSO_4.7H_2O$	0.6 g

Dissolve and make up to 1000 ml with distilled water.

4. Resazurin
Dissolve 100 mg Resazurin in distilled water and make up to 100 ml. Keep refrigerated.

5. Reducing Solution
$Na_2S.H_2O$	373 mg
1 N NaOH	2.6 ml
Distilled water	62 ml

Incubation

Day Before Incubation

Weighing of samples: Weigh 200 ± 10 mg feed samples ground to pass through 1 mm sieve, in a small polypropylene weighing spoon. Fix the weighing spoon containing feed sample to a glass rod with a rubber adaptor and transfer the sample quantitatively, to the closed end of syringe. Weigh each sample in triplicates. With every batch of incubations, have 3 syringes as blank (i.e., without feedstuff), 3 syringes for concentrate reference standard and 3 syringes for roughage reference standard. After weighing of all samples, apply Vaseline to the piston and insert into the syringes. Be careful not to blow the samples out through the nozzle. Clamp the silicone tube fitted to the nozzle. Keep syringes in an incubator or a water bath set at 39°C.

Preparation of Medium (for 60 Incubations)
Distilled water	620 ml
Micromineral Solu.	0.16 ml
Buffer Solu.	310 ml
Macromineral Solu.	310 ml
Resazurin	1.60 ml

Keep in the incubator set at 39°C.

Day of Incubation

1. Keep the medium prepared on the previous day in a water bath set at 39°C, and bubble carbon dioxide slowly for 15 to 20 minutes. Keep the medium continuously stirred with a magnetic stirrer.

2. Collect the rumen fluid from a rumen fistulated animal and prepare as explained (Page 15)
3. Prepare reducing solution and add to the medium. The medium should turn pink and eventually colourless.
4. Measure 650 ml of rumen fluid and add to the medium, continue to bubble carbon dioxide through the medium.
5. Dispense 30 ml rumen inoculum into the syringe through the silicone tube fitted to the nozzle.
6. Push the gas bubbles out, and close the silicone tube with a clamp.
7. Record the volume and put the syringe on the rotor of the incubator or in a water bath set at 39°C.
8. Six to eight hours after incubation, record the reading, unclamp the silicone tube, push the gas out, clamp the tube, record the reading and keep in the incubator.
9. Record the reading again at 24 hours and discard the contents.

Prediction of Digestibility From Gas Production

Gas production recorded from an incubation and calculation of corrected net gas production is presented in Table 2.3.1. Using corrected net gas production and the proximate composition, the ME value of the feedstuff can be predicted with the help of mathematical equations (Menke and Steingass, 1988) (Table 2.3.2)

Table 2.3.1 : Gas Production Data

Sample	Weight (g)	DM (g)	Initial reading ml	Final reading ml	Total gas ml	Net gas ml	Net gas (ml / 200 mg DM)	Corrected net gas ml / 200 mg DM)
Blank	-	-	29	39	8	-		
	-	-	29	36	7	-		
	-	-	29	38	9	-		
				Mean	8			
Concentrate standard	0.2014	0.1813	29	97	68	60	66.2	
	0.2012	0.1771	30	80	50	42	47.4	
	0.2020	0.1818	31	98	67	59	64.9	
						Mean	65.0	
Hay standard	0.2012	0.1771	30	80	50	42	47.4	
	0.2012	0.1771	30	80	50	42	47.4	
	0.2010	0.1769	31	81	50	42	47.5	
						Mean	47.4	

In-Vitro Rumen Studies

Compound feed	0.2046	0.1882	30	80	50	42	44.6	41.3
	0.2049	0.1885	29	80	51	43	45.6	42.2
	0.2032	0.1860	30	79	49	41	43.9	40.6
							Mean	41.4
Wheat straw	0.2011	0.1830	30	62	32	24	26.2	24.3
	0.2005	0.1826	31	62	31	23	25.2	23.3
	0.2003	0.1823	31	63	32	24	26.3	24.3
							Mean	24.0

Calculation of correction factor: Concentrate reference standard should have a net gas production of 60 ml/200 mg DM and hay reference standard 44 ml/200 mg DM.

Therefore, the correction factor for,

Concentrate standard $60/65.0 = 0.9231$

Hay standard $44/47.4 = \dfrac{0.9282}{0.9257}$

The correction factor should be within the range of 0.9 to 1.1. If it falls beyond this range, it is better to discard the incubation. The average of two correction factor is used for correcting net gas production of incubated feed samples.

Equations for Calculation of ME (MJ/Kg) from Gas Production Data:

Concentrates/compound feeds:
$1.06 + 0.157 GP + 0.0084 CP + 0.022 EE - 0.0081 Ash$

Roughages:
$2.20 + 0.1357 GP + 0.0057 CP + 0.0002859 EE^2$

Table 2.3.2 : Calculation of ME content from gas production and chemical composition

	Gas (ml / 200 mg)	CP	EE	Total Ash	ME MJ / kg
		(g per kg dry matter)			
Compound feed	48.6	160	20	70	9.9
Wheat straw	23.9	60	10	120	5.8

The application of these data in diet formulation was examined with straw based diets in lactating dairy cows (Krishnamoorthy et al., 1995; 1998; Nataraja et al., 1998). The observed performance could account for the energy input calculated from the energy value derived by chemical analyses and *in vitro* gas test to the extent of 92%.

Other Applications of *In vitro* Gas Production Technique

Apart from determining dry matter or organic matter digestibility, the possibilities of using *in vitro* rumen studies in other areas - of rumen fermentation have also been explored with variable success. Some examples are the following.

1. Protein degradation and net microbial nitrogen synthesis (Raab *et al.*, 1983).
2. Kinetics of gas production (Blümmel *et al.*, 1990; Krishnamoorthy *et al.*, 1991; Pell and Schoefield, 1993; Groot *et al.*, 1996).
3. Fermentation stoichiometry (Gas, VFAs and microbial biomass) (Blummel, 1994).
4. Interaction between antinutritional factors and rumen fermentation (Khazaal *et al.*, 1994; Makkar *et al.*, 1995; Bhatta *et al.*, 2000).
5. Prediction of dry matter intake and live weight gain from fermentation stoichiometry and kinetics (Khazaal *et al.*, 1993; Blummel *et al.*, 1994).

Chapter 3

IN SITU DACRON BAG STUDIES

Although *in vitro* rumen studies of digestibility determination simulates rumen fermentation to some extent, it is almost impossible to incorporate all dynamics of rumen environment in these techniques. Therefore, the in situ Dacron bag technique was developed as an alternative to the *in vitro* rumen studies (Ørskov and McDonald, 1979). This technique involves placement of feedstuffs in bags made of indigestible fabrics such as nylon, Dacron or silk, directly in the rumen. The loss of dry matter or of any feed component after specific incubation period are measured gravimetrically to determine the rate and extent of degradation.

This technique is widely used, but the procedure differ among the laboratories. Improved methods utilise bags of specific pore size and control the ratio of sample weight to surface area of the bag. Bags with a large ratio of surface area to sample size minimise the error. Optimum pore size is about 40 microns. Smaller pore size retards the entry of organisms and thus inhibit optimum fermentation while larger ones permit transit of lignified particles.

Principle

The dry matter/crude protein disappearance from feeds in polyester bags incubated in the rumen at varying intervals of time are quantitatively determined. These values are used to calculate rapidly degraded, slow degraded, rate of degradation of slow degraded and indigestible fractions. By integrating rate of degradation with the rate of passage, the effective degradability is estimated.

Dry matter/crude protein disappearing at 0.1 hour of incubation is regarded as soluble fraction and hence rapid degraded fraction. Fraction disappearing between 0.1 hour and 48 hour of incubation, as slow degraded fraction and residual at 48 hours or longer is regarded as indigestible fraction,. The rate of disappearance between 0.1 hour and 48 hours is calculated.

Feeding management of the cannulated cow: The degradability of dry matter/protein is an interaction of the intrinsic property of the feed and the rumen environment in which it is fermented. Since the feed offered to the animal can change the rumen environment, it is necessary to have an uniform feeding management of the cannulated cow. This would minimise the interlaboratory variations in the degradability due to varying rumen environment. The feeding management, feed composition and feeding schedule of the cannulated cow should be clearly described when the degradability estimates are published.

Materials Required

Dacron Bags (Fig 3.1) : Earlier work employed use of nylon fabric to stitch bags. Presently Dacron polyester is used. This has the advantage of containing no nitrogen. The bag porosity influences the efflux of feed particles and the permeability of the microbes into the bags. Although a porosity of 35 to 70 microns has gained acceptance it is ideal to use bags of pore size of 35 to 50 microns. Dacron bags can be reused for several incubations provided bags are not damaged and the pore size remains unchanged. Pore size of the bags can be measured using a micrometer under the microscope. The relationship of the sample size (weight) to bag surface area (size) is critical because it influences the nitrogen disappearance. The bags of size 17 cm x 9 cm can be used to incubate 5 g of sample. It is necessary to sew bags using double line stitches with a nylon thread and to have a round base to avoid accumulation of the test feed. This also facilitates easy removal of the residues.

Anchor Weights (Fig. 3.1.) : The position of the bags in the rumen affect digestibility of feedstuffs incubated. Wide variations in digestibility of feeds have been observed when the bags were suspended at different levels in the rumen. In order to avoid floating of the bags on the top of the rumen, it is necessary to attach a weight to anchor bags in the ventral sac of the rumen, where digestion is more rapid. An anchor weight of about 450 g can be made using a strong plastic pipe (10 cm length and 5 cm diameter) filled with concrete. The bags are secured on the anchor weight using a fish line ring. Fish line ring can be made using 20 cm long fish line wire with two ends of the wire tied with a non-slipping barrel knot. The anchor weight is secured to a hook fitted on the cannula using 50 cm long plastic string, which allows free movement of the bag in the rumen.

In-Situ Dacron Bag Studies

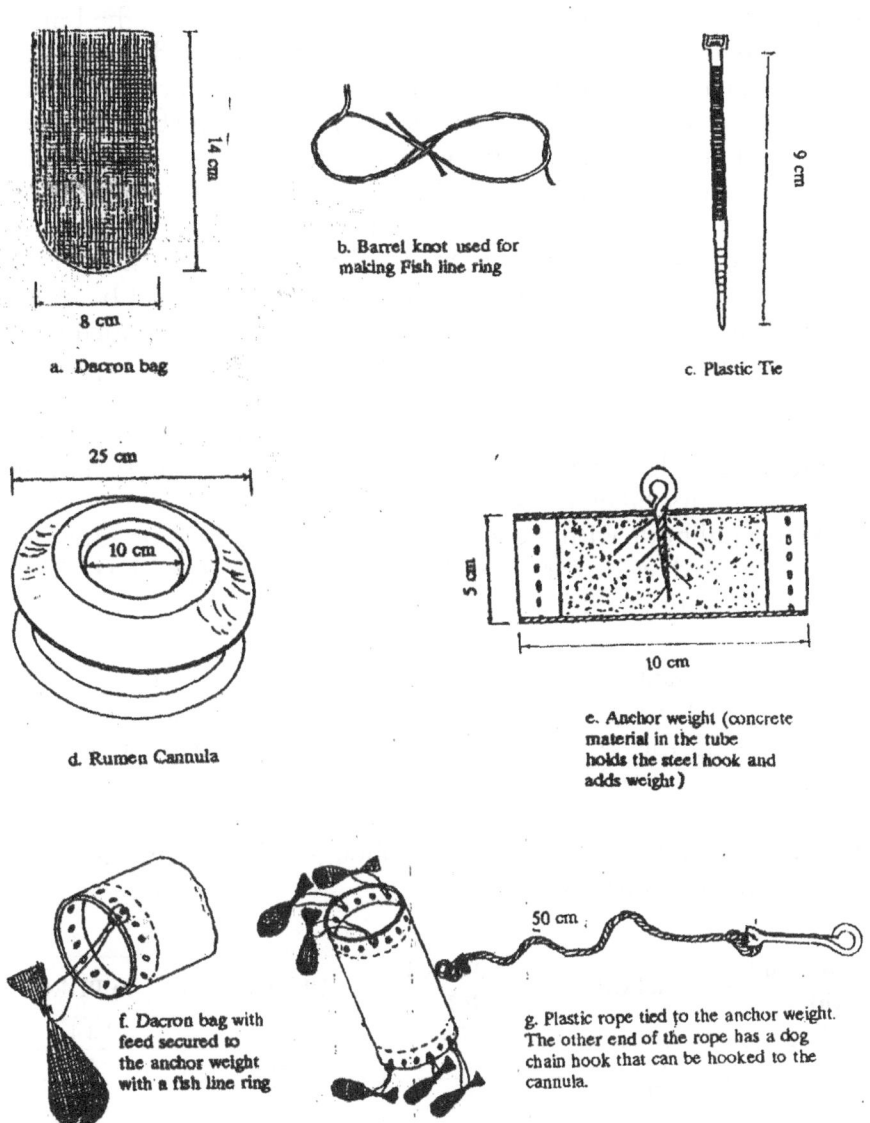

Fig. 3.1 : Materials require for *in situ* rumen incubation

Incubation of Samples in the Rumen : A schematic representation of the incubation of feeds in the rumen is presented in Fig. 3.2. The required number of bags will be washed and dried to a constant weight at 100°C. About 5 g of sample (ground to pass a 3 mm screen) is weighed into the bag and closed with a plastic tie. The bag is then secured to the weight using a plastic loop as illustrated. The bag is then suspended in the rumen by tieing the string to the hook of the cannula. Forage and byproduct feeds will be incubated in the rumen for 0.1, 1, 3, 6, 12, 24, 48, 96 and 168 hours. Concentarte ingredients can be incubated for 0.1, 1, 3, 6, 12, 24, 48 and 72 hours. For each time incubation triplicates are preferred. Thus, twenty four to twenty seven bags are required to complete incubation of one sample. At the end of incubation period, the bags will be removed from the rumen and washed. For the sake of convenience, the incubation is followed in the reverse order; that is, first incubate 148 hour bag followed by 96, 48, 24, 12, 6, 3, 1, and 0.1 so that, all the bags can be removed at once from the rumen and washed. The bags may be rinsed in a washing machine for 2 cycles, each cycle of 5 minutes. The bags are then dried at 60°C for 48 hours, taken out from hot air oven and spread on a table and allowed to equilibrate with the room temperature for 24 hours. The weight of bags with dried residue are recorded. Suitable aliquots of the residue are used to analyse for any desired component of the dry matter.

Example : The data of dry matter and protein degradation studies in cottonseed meal using dacron bag incubations *in situ* are presented in Table 3.1. Using These data, rate and extent of protein degradation can be calculated as illustrated below.

Table 3.1 : Residual crude protein obtained from cottonseed meal incubated in dacron bag *in situ*.

Incubation (h)	Residual CP %	Solubilised CP %	PDRCP	In PDRCP
1	70	30	64	4.16
3	66	34	60	4.09
6	50	50	44	3.78
12	36	64	30	3.40
18	28	72	22	3.09
24	19	81	13	2.56
36	12	88	6	1.79
48	9	91	3	1.10
60	6	94	0	-
72	6	94	0	-

*PDRCP = Potentially digestible residual crude protein.

In-Situ Dacron Bag Studies

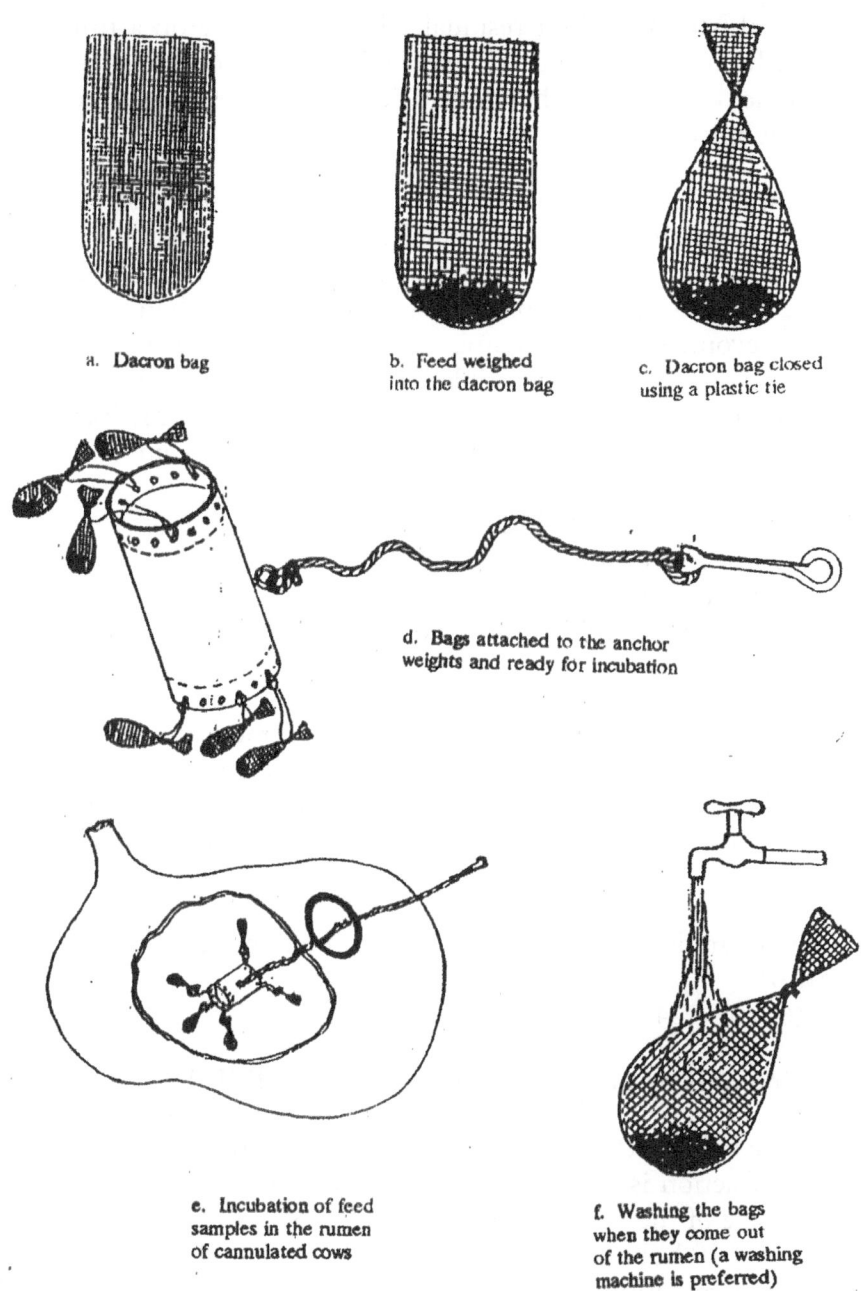

Fig. 3.2 : *In situ* incubation of feed samples in the rumen of cannulated cow

Determination of Rate of Degradation (Kd)

1. Graphical Method : Plot residual CP against time on a three cycle semilogarithmic graph paper (Figure 3.3). A lack of linearity in CP disappearance curve reflects heterogenicity of feed proteins with reference to their solubility characteristics.

(i) Indigestible CP (Fraction C) : An estimate of indigestible CP is obtained from incubations beyond which the residual CP does not decrease any further or decrease marginally. This can be done by extrapolation of residual CP of the terminal one or two incubations (when samples are incubated beyond 48 hours) to time $t = \infty$. The residual CP at a time $t = \infty$ represents an estimate of indigestible CP. Since this fraction is assumed to be indigestible, a rate of digestion of (0%) is assigned to this fraction. In cottonseed meal 72 hour residual CP is considered as an estimate of fraction C.
Potentially digestible CP (PDCP)
PDCP = 100 - Fraction C
    i.e., 100 - 6 = 94
PDCP includes both rapidly degraded (Fraction A) and slowly degraded (Fraction B) protein fractions.

(ii) Slow degraded fraction (Fraction B) : Subtract 'Fraction C' from residual CP obtained at times t, where I = 1 to n, and plot against the corresponding time (Fig. 3.3.). Draw a best fit linear line and extrapolate to time t = 0. The intercept, at time t = 0 is an estimate of the size of fraction B (70%).

(iii) Rapid degraded fraction (Fraction A): Total protein - (Fraction C + Fraction B)
= 100 - (6+70) = 24

Calculation of Rate of Degradation of Fraction B (Kd)

(i) Calculate half life ($t\frac{1}{2}$) of Fraction B. Half life is the time at which the size of the fraction is reduced by one half. In Fig.3.3. $t\frac{1}{2}$ is the time at which the size of the Fraction B is reduced to 35% from the initial 70%.
        ($t\frac{1}{2}$ = 10 hours).
(ii) Rate of degradation (kd) = $0.693/t\frac{1}{2}$
                            = 0.693/10
                            = 0.0693 h-1 (6.93%/hr)

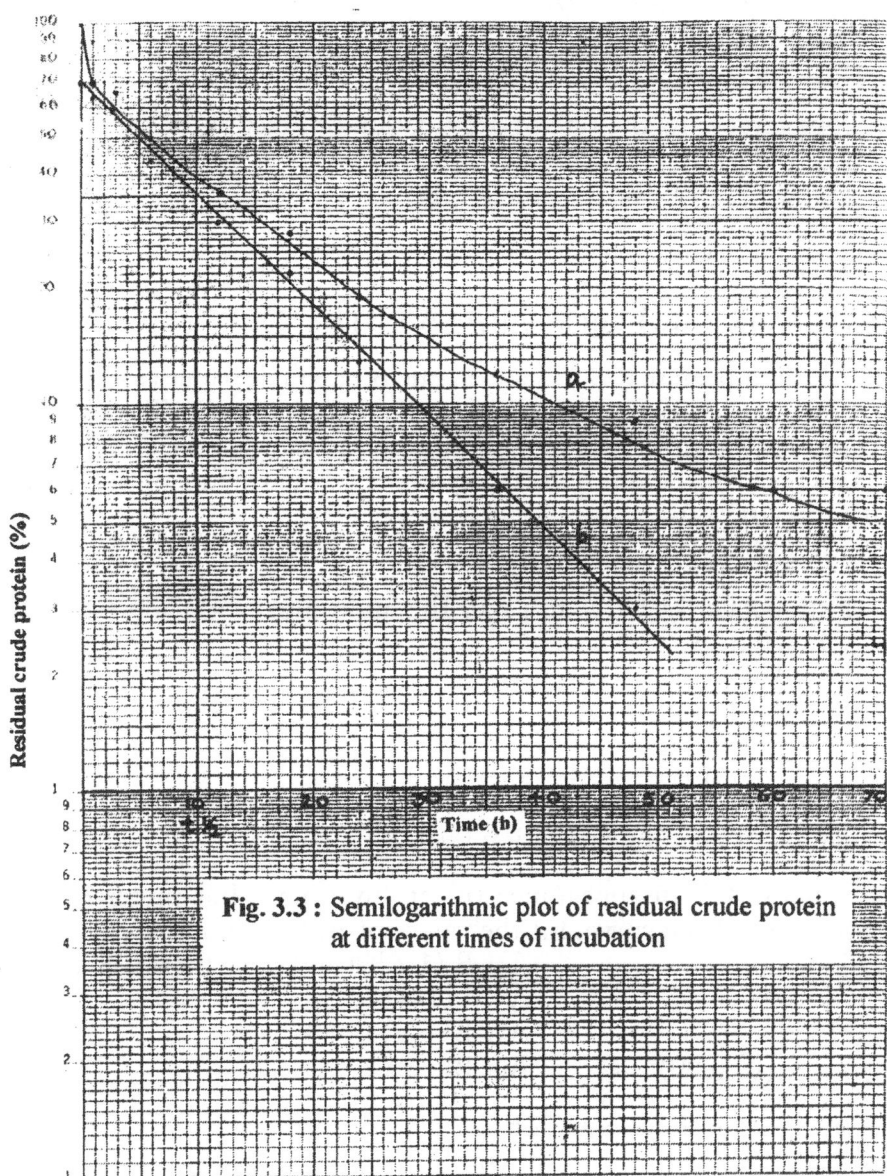

Fig. 3.3 : Semilogarithmic plot of residual crude protein at different times of incubation

2. Regression Method : Rate of degradation of fraction B can also be calculated by regression of natural log (ln) of PDRCP against time. The inv. ln of intercept represents size of fraction B and the slope represents rate of degradation. From the data presented in Table 3.1, the regression of ln PDRCP against time resulted in

$\hat{Y} = 4.22 - 0.0662 \times (r\ 0.999)$.
 Therefore, Fraction B = Inv. ln 4.22
 = 68

The slope represents the rate of degradation of Fraction B. Therefore, kd =0.0662
Fraction A = PDRCP - Fraction B
 = 94 - 68
 = 26

3. Using Exponential Equation: $p = A + B(1-e^{-kdt})$

Plot CP disappearance (%) against time on a graph paper (Figure 3.4.). Asympote of the curve represents potentially digestible CP. Therefore, CP disappearance at time $t = \infty$ represents potentially digestible CP (Fraction A + Fraction B). Therefore, 100 - asympote, is an estimate of Fraction C.
PDRCP = 100 - 04
 = 6%

Extrapolate the curve to $t = 0$. The intercept at $t = 0$, represents the size of Fraction A.
Fraction A = 24
Fraction B = PDRCP - A
 = 94 - 24
 = 70 %

Calculation of rate of degradation (kd) of Fraction B:

Choose CP disappearance (p) at any time t, but preferably at a sensitive area of the curve. Fit the values of A, B, p and t in exponential equation,

$p = A + B(1-e^{-kdt})$ and solve for kd as follows:
$p = A + B(1-e^{-kdt})$
$p = A + B - (B)(e^{-kdt})$
$(B)(e^{-kdt}) = A + B - p$

Rearranging the above equation,

$$e^{-kdt} = \frac{A + B - p}{B}$$

Taking natural log e on both sides of the equation, we have
Rearranging the above equation,

$$\ln(e^{-kdt}) = \ln \frac{A + B - p}{B}$$

$$^{-kdt} \ln e = \ln \frac{A + B - p}{B}$$

$$^{-kdt} (1) = \ln \frac{A + B - p}{B}$$

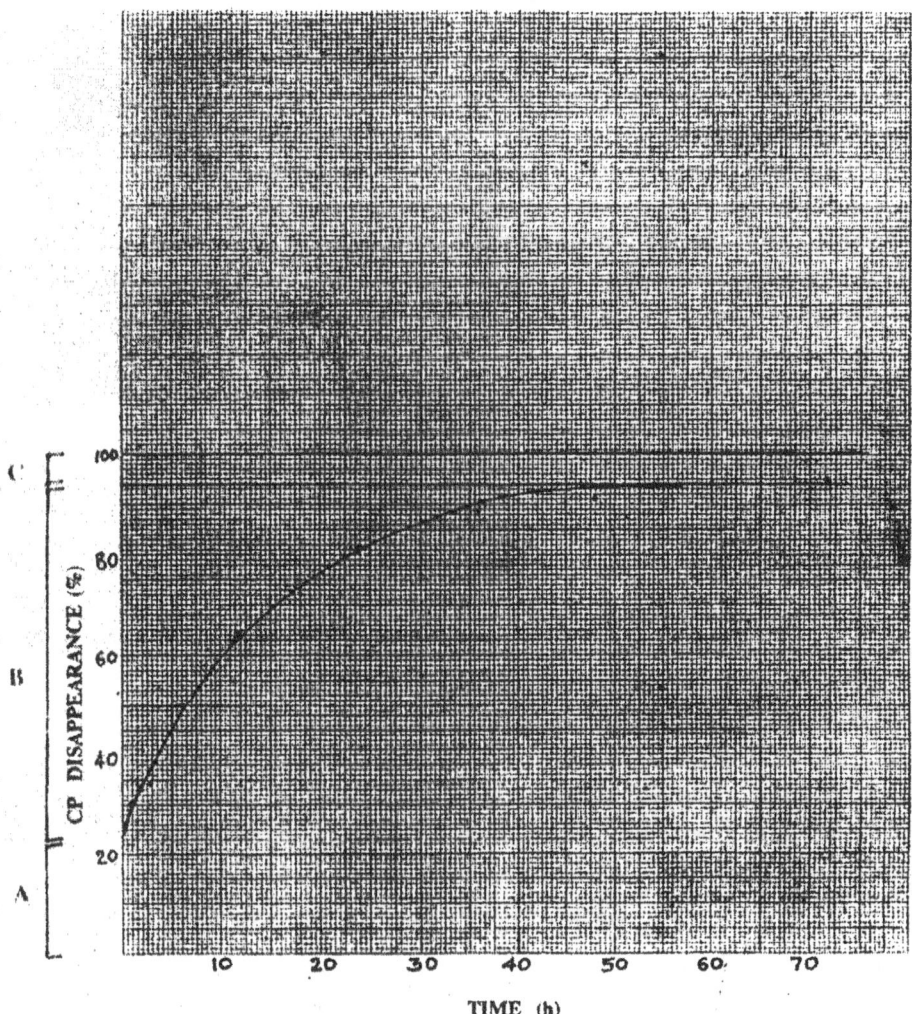

Fig. 3.4 : Crude protein disappearance from Dacron bags at different times of incubation

Example : Let us consider p at 10 hour. At 10 hour, solubilised CP is 60 (Fig. 3.4.).

Therefore, $e^{-kdt(10)} = \ln \frac{24 + 70 - 60}{70}$

$(10) (k_d) \ln e = \ln \dfrac{24 + 70 - 60}{70}$

$10_{kd} (1) = \ln (.4857)$
$10_{kd} = 0.7222$
$k_d = -0.7222/10$
$k_d = 0.0722$

4. Using Computer Programme

The Dacron bag data on dry matter and protein disappearance can also be analysed by using computer programmes. The data presented in Table 3.1. is analysed by using the programme developed at the Rowett Research Institute, Aberdeen, U.K. The output of the results obtained are presented below.

Model based on McDonald 1981 *J.Agric.Sci.Camb.* **96:** 251 -252

The Degradation Curve Is Described As:
1. Within a lag time   T = A i.e. the initial washing loss.
2. Beyond the time   T = a+b (1-e^{-ct})

Potential degradation (B) is calculated as a+b-A

Cottonseed meal (Data in Table 3.1)
A   =   24.34 Washing loss is not measured
The value for A is taken as the fitted value as in the curve.
B   =   70.13
A+B   =   94.47
C   =   0.0672
    Lag time T = .0 hr

The Fitted Curve Is:
Y   =   24.34 + 70.13 [1-e$^{(-0.0672t)}$]
RSD   =   1.74

Times	1	3	6	12	18	24	36	48	60	72
Measurements	30.00	34.00	50.00	64.00	72.00	81.00	88.00	91.00	94.00	94.00
Fitted values	28.90	37.15	47.62	63.18	73.56	80.50	88.24	91.69	93.23	93.92
Rumen outflow rate (k)			.0100	.0200	.0300	.0400	.0500	.0600		
A+b*c/(c+k)* EXP (-(c+K)*T)			85.4	78.4	72.8	68.3	64.6	61.4		
Rumen outflow rate (k)			.0700	.0800	.0900	.1000	.1100	.1200		
A+b*c/(c+k)* EXP (-(c+k)*T)			58.7	56.4	54.3	52.5	50.9	49.5		

Determination of Effective Degradability (P)

The extent of degradability of any feed component in the rumen is a function of rate of degradation and rate of passage. Fraction A, or the soluble faction is assumed to be degraded almost instantaneously and Fraction C or the indigestible fraction is assumed to be not degraded. Therefore, the degradation rate, kd, applied to Fraction B, which must be related to rate of passage.

The effective degradability (P) of any feed component can be derived by the equation,

$$P = A + B [k_d /(k_p + k_d)]$$

Where, P = effective degradability, A = soluble fraction, B = insoluble degradable fraction, kd = rate of degradation of B, and kp = rate of passage. A, B and kd are constants derived from the exponential equation $p = A + B (1-e^{-kdt})$ describing degradation. The outflow rates for protein supplements are reported to vary from 0.01/h at maintenance level of intake to 0.1/h at higher level of feeding.

Calculation of P For Different Fractional Outflow Rates:

Fraction A = 30
B = 64
Kd = 0.068
Kp = 0.03, 0.06, 0.09
P   = $A+B[K_d/K_p+K_d]$
K_p 0.03 0.06 0.09
P(%)   74.4 64.0 57.5

Thus, the same feedstuff can have different effective degradability depending upon the rate of passage, which is influenced by factors such as level of intake, particle size, roughage to concentrate ratio etc.

Chapter 4

NITROGEN FRACTIONATION BY CHEMICAL AND *IN VITRO* METHODS

Although the Dacron bag technique for protein degradation measurement is relatively simple and not too expensive as compared to *in vivo* measurements, the technique is not easily adaptable in laboratories that are not fully equipped to maintain cannulated animals. Therefore, different alternative approaches such as measurement of protein solubilities in buffer, enzymes and detergent solutions have been tried (Pichard and Van Soest, 1978; Krishnamoorthy et al., 1982, 1983, 1995; Aufrere et al.,1991; Prabhu *et al.*, 1996; Licitra et al., 1996 and 1998). The advantages of these approaches are that, they are simple, rapid, economical and repeatable. However, since the enzymes used are not of rumen microbial origin, degradation obtained from these enzymes may not be a true .reflection of degradation occurring in the rumen. Nevertheless, because of their simplicity and rapidity, in situations where large number of samples are to be compared, *in vitro* techniques serve as useful tools.

Buffer Insoluble Nitrogen (BIN)

Based on the observations that the solubility of proteins is a predisposing factor for degradation by rumen microorganisms, soluble N has been suggested as an estimate of rapidly degraded N. However, soluble N does not provide an estimate of rumen degraded N because variable amounts of insoluble N can also undergo rapid degradation in the rumen. Nitrogen insoluble in borate phosphate buffer is regarded as buffer insoluble nitrogen.

Protease Insoluble Nitrogen (PIN)

The amount of nitrogen degraded in the rumen is influenced by the physicochemical nature of the feed N, proteolytic activity of rumen fluid and retention time of the protein in the rumen. The degraded nitrogen in the feedstuffs could be estimated through integration of the rate of passage and rate of degradation. Therefore, it is difficult to obtain as precise estimate of rumen degraded N for a given feedstuff from any *in vitro* technique without an accurate knowledge of rumen proteolytic activity and rate of passage of feed N. However, to evaluate feedstuffs on a relative basis an *in vitro* procedure using protease from *Streptomyces griseus* (Pichard and Van Soest, 1978; Krishnamoorthy et al., 1983) has been proposed to determine the rumen degraded N and undegraded N. Nitrogen insoluble in protease enzyme is regarded as rumen undegradable N.

Acid Detergent Insoluble Nitrogen (ADIN)

Nitrogen contained in ADF is termed acid detergent insoluble N (ADIN) and is comprised of the N fraction of the lignin, Maillard reaction products and tannin-protein complexes. ADIN is negatively correlated with N digestibility and it can be used as an estimate of indigestible N in feedstuffs (Van Soest, 1994).

Procedures

The procedures used for feed N evaluation for ruminants *in vitro* are variable with different group of researchers. It is rather difficult to recommend any procedure as a standard. However, the procedures that we are using currently in India are presented below.

4.1 Buffer insoluble nitrogen (Krishnamoorthy *et al.*, 1982; Licitra *et al.*, 1996)

Reagents:
1. Borate phosphate buffer: pH 6.8: $NaH_2PO_4H_2O$, 12.2 g/L; $Na_2BO_410H_2O$, 8.91 g/L
2. t-butyl alcohol, 10%: 10ml t-butyl alcohol in distilled water made up to 100 ml.

Procedure:
- Grind feed sample to pass 1 mm sieve.
- Weigh 0.5±0.1 g sample into a 100 ml beaker.
- Add 5 ml of 10% t-butyl alcohol and mix with a glass rod.

- Add 25 ml borate phosphate buffer, pH 6.8 and stir thoroughly.
- Add another 25 ml borate phosphate buffer, and leave it for one hour.
- Filter the contents of the beaker through Whatman No. 54 filter paper using mild vacuum suction.
- Wash the residue with about 300 ml distilled water.
- Remove the filter paper with the residue and estimate N by Kjeldahl method to obtain the insoluble N content of the feedstuff.
- Calculate the soluble N content as the difference between total N and buffer insoluble N.

(The true protein and non-protein nitrogen components of soluble protein can also be determined by tungstic acid and trichloracetic acid precipitation procedures described in Licitra *et al.*, 1996)

4.2 Protease Insoluble Nitrogen (Krishnamoorthy *et al.*, 1983; Licitra *et al.*, 1998)

Reagents:
1. **Borate Phosphate Buffer :** pH 7.8-8.0; $NaH_2PO_4H_2O$, 7.6g/L, $Na_2B_4O_7.10H_2O$, 13.17g/L.
2. **Protease Solution :** (Protease from type XIV *Streptomyces griseus* (Sigma Chemical Co., St. Louis). Prepare an enzyme concentration of 330 x 10^{-3} units/ml in borate phosphate buffer. Filter through Whatman No. 54 filter paper. Use filtrate for incubation.

Procedure:
- Weigh 0.5g of air dry sample (ground through 1 mm screen) in 125 ml Erlenmeyer flask)
- Add 40 ml borate phosphate buffer (7.8-8.0 pH).
- Keep in water bath at 39°C for 1 h.
- Add 10 ml of protease solution.
- Keep in water bath for 18 h (concentrates) or 48 h (roughages).
- Filter through Whatman No. 54 filter paper using vacuum suction.
- Wash the residue using 250 ml distilled water.
- Transfer the residue along with filter paper into a kjeldahl flask and determine the N.
- Rumen undegraded N is calculated as (N in the residue/Total N incubated) x 100

Modified procedure of protein degradability — Licitra *et al.*, 1998

The procedure of protein degradability (Krishnamoorthy *et al.*,1983) has been modified and proposed by Licitra et al. (1998). In this procedure 6.7

pH buffer was preferred. The amount of units of enzyme (UE) used was fixed at a constant ratio to the true protein (TP) content (13.4 UE/TP) by keeping constant the sample weight (0.5 g) and varying the amount of protease solution (using a concentration of 0.33 UE/ml protease solution). The TP content in feeds was determined by tungstic acid precipitation (Refer Licitra et al., 1996). The standard incubation times were reduced from 48 h to 30 h for the forages and to 24 h for corn silages and byproducts with high content of NDF.

The fixed ratio of units of enzyme/TP (13.4) was calculated by considering the amount of TP contained in 0.5 g of soybean meal on DM basis. Therefore, 0.5 g of soybean meal with 54.8% CP/DM, and 49.3% TP/DM received 3.3 UE in 10 ml of protease solution (0.33 UE/ml); the amount of TP in 0.5 g of soybean meal is equal to 0.5 x 49.3 = 0.246 TP/DM, and the fixed ratio was calculated as 3.3/0.246 = 13.4 UE/TP. The amount of protease solution can be defined for every feed, for example in Brewer's grain containing 24.6% CP and 23.5% TP on DMB; The TP of Brewers grain was divided by standard TP of Soybean meal and multiplied with standard amount of protease solution (23.5/49.3) x 10 = 4.77 ml of protease solution. Therefore, (4.77 x 0.33 =) 1.574 units of enzyme was used on 0.118 g of TP in brewers grain.

4.3 Acid Detergent Insoluble Nitrogen (Goering and Van Soest, 1970)

Please refer Page 10.

Table 4.2.1: Biological significance of chemical / *in vitro* fractions of feed nitrogen

Nitrogen fraction	Biological significance
Acid detergent insoluble N (ADIN)	Estimate of unavailable N
Total N-ADIN	Estimate of total available N
Protease insoluble N (PIN)	Estimate of total rumen undergraded N
PIN — ADIN	Estimate of available rumen undergraded N
Buffer insoluble N (BIN)	Pooled estimate of slow rumen degradable, available rumen undergraded and unavailable N
Total N — BIN	Estimate of rapid solubilisable N (includes soluble NPN and soluble true protein)
BIN — PIN	Estimate of slow rumen solubilisable N (mainly proteins requiring proteolytic enzyme for solubilistaion)

•••

Chapter 5

ENZYMATIC METHODS

Different enzymatic methods have been proposed as potential alternatives to rumen inoculum studies to determine dry matter digestibility and protein degradation. However, the type of enzyme used and the procedure adopted differ (Marten and Barnes, 1979). The enzyme methods offer distinct advantage under circumstances of the difficulties in maintaining rumen fistulated animals as a source of rumen inoculum. Since, the enzymes used in these techniques are commercially available enzyme preparations, and are not of rumen microbial origin, the digestibility obtained from these techniques are related to *in vivo* digestibility by means of mathematical equations. Therefore, equations developed to predict energy content using enzyme techniques differ with the type of feedstuff and type of enzymes used in the technique (Table 5.1.) (Martens and Barnes, 1979). The enzyme methods are popular among the feed compounding industries to evaluate raw materials and compound feeds.

The method used by DeBoever *et al.* (1986) to determine digestibility of mixed feeds is given below.

5.1 Pepsin-HCl-Cellulase Method Of Estimating DOMDM (De Boever *et al.*, 1986)

Reagents
1. Pepsin hydrochloric acid solution: Dissolve 2 g pepsin (Merck No. 7190, 1:10,000) in 0.1 M HCl.
2. Cellulase-buffer solution
2.1 Acetate buffer pH 4.8 (0.1 M) - Dilute 5.9 ml acetic acid (CH_3COOH, 96%) with water to 1 litre (Solution A).

Dissolve 13.6 g sodium acetate ($CH_3COONa\ 3\ H_2O$) in water and make the volume up to 1 litre (Solution B).
Mix 400 ml of solution A with 600 ml of solution B and control pH. Increase in pH results from the addition of solution B, decrease from the addition of solution A.

2.2   Cellulase enzyme - Onozuka (*Trichoderma viridae*) R-10 (Maruzen Chem Co., Japan): Dissolve 3.3 g in 1 litre buffer.

Procedure
1. An air dry sample (1 mm) of 0.3 g is weighed to the nearest mg into a sintered glass crucible (capacity 50 ml porosity 1) provided with a screw cap at the bottom.
2. Add 30 ml of preheated pepsin-HCl solution. Close the top with plastic film, place the crucible in an incubator at 40°C for 24 hours. After 5 hours stir the contents.
3. Transfer the crucible into a water bath set at 80°C for exactly 45 minutes. Filter and rinse the contents with warm water.
4. Add 30 ml of preheated cellulase-buffer mixture (with bottom side closed). Close the top and place in the incubator for 24 hours at 40°C. Stir after 5 hours.
5. Filter, wash with warm water, dry overnight at 103°C. Cool and weigh. Ignite in a muffle furnace at 550°C for 1.5 hour. Cool and weigh again.
6. Subtracting percentage of indigestible organic matter from 100, gives cellulase digestibility of the organic matter (CDOM). The cellulase digestible organic matter in the dry matter (CDOMD) is calculated by multiplying CDOM by the content of organic matter in dry matter).

CDOMD measured by this technique was better correlated with the *in vivo* DOMD of 40 compound feeds varying between 0.59 and 0.90 than was the *in vitro* DOMD following Tilley and Terry (1963). The results also showed that cellulase method is more repeatable than the *in vitro* method.

5.2 Use of Protease (*Streptomyces griseus*) Enzyme to Determine Protein Degradation In The Rumen

Enzymatic methods to determine protein degradation in the rumen has received much attention in the recent years (Nocek, 1988). The most often used enzyme in this technique is the protease from *Streptomyces* griseus (Pichard and VanSoest, 1977; Krishnamoorthy *et al*., 1983; Aufrere *et al*., 1991; Licitra *et al*., 1998 and Prabhu *et a*l., 1998).

Determination of protein degradability using protease from Streptomyces griseus (Krishnamoorthy *et al*., 1983; Licitra *et al*., 1998). Refer Section 4.2, Page 29.

Table 5.1: Equations for predicting dry matter digestibility (%) in feedstuffs from enzymatic methods (Martens and Barnes, 1979)

Reference	Forage type	Primary type of digestion	Correlation with *in vivo* or *in vitro*	Prediction equation (y=% *in vitro* DMD x=% enzyme DMD)	Error expression
Jones & Hayward (1973)	Temperate grasses	Cellulose	0.92 (*vivo*)	Y=0.72x+33.0	RSD 2.5
Pulli (1976)	Temperate grasses	Cellulose (Jones & Hayward, 1973)	0.99(*vitro*)	-	RSD 1.3
	Grass and Red clover		0.99(*vitro*)	-	RSD 0.9
Dowman & Collins (1977)	Grass silage	Cellulose (Modified Jones & Hayward 1973	0.89 (*vivo*)	Y=0.58x+31.6 (organic matter)	RSD 2.3
McQueen & Van Soest (1975)	Temperate grasses & Legumes	Cellulose + hemicellulase	0.80 (*vivo*)	-	SE 6.0
Jones & Hayward (1975)	Temperate grasses	Pepsin + cellulose	0.96 (*vivo*)	Y=0.61x+30.4	RSD 2.4
	Temperate legumes		0.94 (*vitro*)	Y=0.60x+31.6	RSD 2.7
Adegbola & Paladines (1977)	Tropical Grasses & Legumes	Pepsin + cellulose (Jones & Haywards 1975)	0.98 (*vivo*)	-	S_{yx} 2.3
Goto & Minson (1977)	Tropical & temperate grasses	Pepsin + cellulose (Modified Jones & Haywards 1975)	0.94 (*vivo*)	Y=0.69x+20.3	RSD 2.7
Terry *et al.*, (1978)	Tropical and temperate grasses	Pepsin + cellulose (Goto & Minson 1977)	0.94 (*vivo*)	Y=0.56x+34.7	RSD 1.8
McLeod & Monson (1979)	Tropical & temperate grasses	Pepsin + cellulose (Goto & Minson 1977)	0.94 (*vivo*)	Y=0.70x+18.2	RSD 2.6
	Tropical & Temperate Legumes		0.91 (*vivo*)	Y=0.60x+22.2	RSD 3.1
Roughman & Holland (1977)	Temperate grasses & legumes	Neutral detergent fibre + cellulose	0.98 (*vivo*)	Y=0.98x-10.12	RSD 2.8

Chapter 6

HOHENHEIM GAS TEST- OTHER APPLICATIONS

6.1 Kinetics of Rumen Digestion

The rate and extent of digestion of dry matter or organic matter in the rumen is regarded as the important parameter to predict voluntary feed intake (Khazaal *et al.*, 1993; Blummel,1994). Voluntary feed intake is responsible for more than 50 per cent of the variations in animal response to the diet (Van Soest, 1994) and with low quality unsupplemented roughages, this can be as much as 93% (Blumme1,1994). Therefore, any parameter of feed evaluation that would indicate the voluntary feed intake would be a useful parameter to judge the quality of feedstuff. The rate of digestion of any feed component can be measured by determining extent of digestion at intervals of time. Therefore, the techniques for determining extent of digestion, such as the rumen *in vitro* techniques (Tilley and Terry, 1963; Goering and Van Soest, 1970) or the *in situ* Dacron bag technique have been adopted to derive rate of degradation of dry matter of any particular component of the feedstuff. However, unlike in determining the extent of digestion, wherein the incubation is turned off at one particular time (normally 48 hours), measurement of rate of digestion, requires termination of incubation at several points between the start of incubation and until at least 90% of the potentially digestible dry matter is digested (72 or 96 hours). This generates a large number of samples for analysis.

In gas production technique, since gas produced from digestion of substrate is accumulated in the incubations, measurement of gas at different times of incubation would reflect the extent of digestion at different times of incubation. Therefore, unlike with other *in vitro* / *in situ* techniques wherein, digestion is determined from the gravimetric disappearance of feed at different times of incubation, gas production technique offers the possibility of using cumulative gas production at different times of incubation to measure the rate of digestion. Thus, a single incubation of feedstuffs is adequate to measure the rate of gas production.

Procedure

The preparations and procedure for incubation are explained in section 2.3. (page 17) with the following modifications.
- Continue the incubations up to 96 hours
- Record gas production at 2, 4, 6, 8, 12, 16, 24, 36, 48, 56, 72, and 96 hours.
- Evacuate the syringes and reset to 30 ml when the reading exceeds 85 ml.
- Calculate net gas production and determine rate of gas production by means of exponential model (Blummel, 1994) $Y = a+b(1-e^{-ct})$

Where,
Y = cumulative gas production at a given time (ml)
a = rapidly produced (intercept of the equation)
b = gas volume from the insoluble but fetmentable fraction
c = rate of gas production, t = time of fermentation
a+b = potential gas volume or the asymptote of gas production

The experiment conducted with a large number of cereal straws have indicated a close relationship between *in vitro* gas production parameters and voluntary feed consumption (Table 5.1) (Blummel, 1994).

Table 6.1 : Correlation (R2) between parameters a, b, (a+b) and c of *in vitro* gas
production and the dry matter intake of cereal straws

Parameter	R2	P
a+b+c	0.747	0.0001
B	0.462*	0.0001
A	0.220*	0.0001
C	0.065*	0.0007
(a+b)+c	0.623	0.0001
A+b	0.601*	0.0001
C	0.022*	0.0850

Therefore, the kinetic parameters of gas production can be used to predict DMI to assess the differences in the quality of straw.

$$\text{DMI g/kg}^{0.75}/d = 25.49 + 1.66a + 0.61b + 332.29c$$

The gas production technique to measure kinetics of fermentation has been further improved by the use of pressure transducers (Theodorou et al., 1993) and automatic recording system (Pell and Schoefield, 1993). The appropriateness of different mathematical models to explain the kinetics have received much attention (Groot et al., 1006; France et al., 1998; Dhanoa et al., 1998).

6.2 Protein Degradation and Microbial Protein Synthesis

The possibilities of using Hohenheim gas test to determine rumen protein degradation and microbial protein synthesis was explored by Raab et al., (1983). When the microbes derive energy (ATPs) from carbohydrate fermentation and produce CO_2, CH_4 and VFAs, nitrogen constituents such as ammonia, amino acids, and peptides derived from protein degradation are incorporated into cell protein. Since degradation of carbohydrates and proteins, and synthesis of microbial protein occur simultaneously, using the mathematical relationship between gas production and ammonia nitrogen disappearance in the incubations, protein degradation and efficiency of microbial protein synthesis can be determined.

Procedure
1. Weigh the samples of test feed to provide 26 mg of crude protein into 100 ml calibrated syringes along with 50, 100, 150 and 200 mg starch or cellulose in triplicates along with rumen inoculum blank.
2. Incubate the feed samples with rumen inoculum as explained before (section 2, page 18) and record the initial reading.
3. At the desired time of terminating incubations, record the readings and place the syringes in an ice bath to stop microbial activity.
4. Transfer the contents of syringes quantitatively to kjeldahl flask and distill ammonia.
5. Regress ammonia nitrogen (mg) against gas volume and calculate the intercept (ammonia nitrogen at zero gas production) and slope.
6. Calculate protein degraded as follows.

$$\% \text{ IVDN} = \frac{\text{Ammonia nitrogen at zero gas production - ammonia nitrogen of blank}}{\text{Total nitrogen of feedstuff incubated}}$$

7. The slope of regression line of ammonia nitrogen against gas volume is the net ammonia incorporation into the cells indicating the efficiency of microbial nitrogen synthesis.

6.3 Interference of Antinutritional Components in Rumen Digestion

A wide variety of antinutritional components are distributed in tropical plants. Since, the chemical nature of these compounds are too diverse, determination of these constituents by chemical analyses would be too expensive and further they do not indicate the extent of their interference in the process of rumen digestion. This is particularly true for heterogenous group of compounds such as tannins, saponins, alkaloids, etc. When these components are solubles, techniques involving gravimetric determination of digestibility (*in vitro* and *in situ*) would regard these constituents as nutritionally available. Therefore, suitability of such techniques to evaluate feedstuffs that contain soluble antinutritional components is questionable. Since, gas production is an *in vitro* technique reflects both microbial growth (Krishnamoorthy *et al.*, 1991; Beuvink, 1993) and feed character (Blümmel *et al.*, 1994; Beuvink, 1993; Steingass and Menke, 1988) the posiibilities of using gas production measurement to assess the interference of antinutritional components in the process of rumen digestion have been explored (Beuvink, 1993; Khazaal *et al.*, 1994; Makkar *et al.*, 1995). The use of gas test to study the influence of tanniferous feedstuffs on rumen fermentation process has received much attention in the recent years. Certain types of tannins and saponins at low concentration have been reported to slow down the rate of gas production, and increase the microbial efficiency without affecting the total gas production (Makkar et al., 1995). The extent of interference of tannins on digestion of feedstuffs can be assessed by the increase in gas production consequent to addition of polyethylene glycol (PEG) 6000 (Makkar *et al.*, 1995 Jamuna *et. al.*, 2012). This approach has been used to assess the interference of tannins present in Bengal gram husk and Tamarind seed husk in rumen fermentation of carbohydrates (Sreerangaraju et al., 2000; Bhatta et al., 2000) and microbial nitrogen synthesis. Since PEG binds with tannins and results in increased gas production, the magnitude of increase is suggestive of the degree of tannin interference in nutrient digestion in the rumen. From the results published in the literature, it appears that the gas production technique has a good potential to study the influence of antinitritional components present in feedstuffs on the process of rumen digestion.

Determination of Extent of Interference of Tannins in Rumen Digestion of Feedstuffs

Reagents
1. Same as those required for gas test
2. Polyethyleneglycol (PEG) 6000

Procedure

The preparations and procedure for incubation are explained in section 2 page 18 with the following modifications.

Incubate feed samples without and with PEG 6000 at a ratio of 1:2 (feed : PEG 6000) by weight along with PEG 6000 blank.

Record gas production. The increase in gas production on PEG 6000 addition is an indication of the extent of interference of tannins in ruminal digestion of feedstuffs.

Chapter 7

RUMEN LIQUOR ANALYSIS

Introduction

In ruminants, nutritional studies are very complicated unlike non ruminants where it is quite simple. In non-ruminants, analysis of feed taken and faeces voided by the animal gives overall picture of digestion and nutrient availability to the animal. In ruminants, since it has a complex microbial digestive system (rumen) within the animal digestive system, the analysis of the feed taken and faeces voided will not express the whole processes in the GI tract of the animal. To have complete picture, it is necessary to study at the site of microbial digestion (rumen). For such study, samples from the rumen have to be drawn and analyzed for metabolities, microbial enzymes etc.

Collection of rumen sample and its preservation

1. Rumen liquor samples are drawn from the fistulated animals by probe or by the stomach tube in the intact animals. For biochemical analysis collect the sample in the flask kept in ice bath, but for enzyme estimation rumen liquor collecton should be made at 39°C.
2. Filter the rumen liquor through four layers of muslin cloth (strained rumen liquor).
3. For biochemical analysis 2 drops of 20% H_2SO_4 is added to 20ml of rumen liquor immediately after collection.
4. Acidified samples should be stored at -20°C till analyzed.
5. For enzymatic studies rumen liquor samples should be processed immediately after collection.

(A) Rumen Metabolities

Volatile Fatty Acids (VFA)

Principle

In acidic medium volatile fatty acids remain in the acid form and by heating get vaporized. The vapors of VFA are condensed and titrated against standard alkali in the presence of indicator (Barnett, and Reid, 1956).

Apparatus
1. Balance
2. Markham apparatus
3. Heating mantle
4. Burette
5. Conical flask
6. Pipette
7. Ice bath

Reagents
1. Oxalate buffer
   a) Potassium oxalate 10% - Take 10g potassium oxalate, dissolve it and make the volume to 100 ml with distilled water.
   b) Oxalic acid (5%) - Take 5g oxalic acid, dissolve it and make volume to 100 ml with distilled water.
   c) Mix soln. A and B.
       or
   d) Saturated magnesium sulphate in 1N H_2SO_4
2. 0.01N NaOH
3. Phenolpthalein indicator: 0.1g phenolpthalein, dissolve in 50 ml ethanol and add to it 50 ml distilled water.

Procedure
1. Connect the Markham apparatus with a round bottom flask (2 lit.) half filled with water, kept on heating mantle (Fig. 1).
2. Allow the water to boil.
3. Pipette 2 ml strained rumen liquor and then 2 ml buffer in the apparatus. Wash the funnel with distilled water.
4. Allow the sample to boil.
5. Collect 100 ml distilled VFA in 250 ml flask kept in ice bath.
6. Add few drops of phenolpthalein and titrate the distillate with 0.01N NaOH till pink colour develops (end point).
7. Read the volume of 0.01N NaOH used for titration on the burette.

Calculation

M.equivalent or mmol TVFA/100 ml rumen liquor

$$= \frac{\text{Vol. of NaOH used} \times \text{Strength of NaOH} \times 100}{\text{Vol. of rumen liquor taken}}$$

$$= \frac{\text{Vol. of NaOH used} \times 0.01 \times 100}{2.0}$$

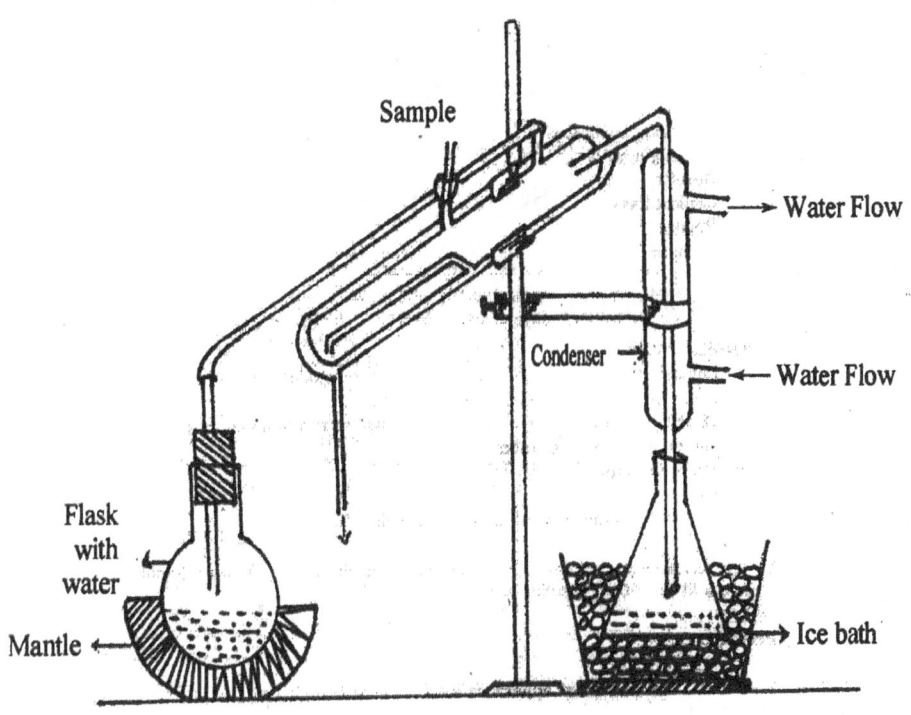

Fig.1 : Markham Apparatus

Precautions
1. Boiling of sample should be very gentle.
2. Distillate should be collected in precooled flask and should be kept in ice bath till titrated. Rise in temperature will result in loss of volatile fatty acids from the distillate.
3. During titration, stiff the contents of the flask continuously.
4. End point is the point where pink color persist atleast for 30 seconds

Total Nitrogen

Principle
When sample containing nitrogen is digested with H_2SO_4, the total nitrogen converts into ammonium sulphate $(NH_4)_2SO_4$. In the presence of alkali, ammonia is released from the ammonium sulphate and released ammonia is distilled and trapped in a known volume of standard acid, which is than back titrated with the standard alkali. The whole process is completed in three steps. The reactions during estimation are as follows

Digestion
Organic nitrogen + Conc. H_2SO_4 = $(NH_4)_2SO_4$

Distillation
$(NH_4)_2SO_4 + 2NaOH = Na_2SO_4 + 2NH_3 + 2H_2O$

Trapping
$2NH_3 + H_2SO_4 = (NH_4)_2SO_4$

Apparatus
1. Balance
2. Micro kjeldahl distillation assembly (Fig. 2)
3. Digestion bench
4. Kjeldahl flasks
5. Pipette
6. Conical flask
7. Beaker
8. Burette
9. Volumetric flask

Reagents
1. Digestion mixture (K_2SO_4 + $CuSO_4$ in the ratio of 9:1): 90g potassium sulphate and 10g copper sulphate mixed together.
2. Concentrated H_2SO_4
3. 40% NaOH solution
4. 0.01N NaOH
5. 0.01N H_2SO_4
6. Methyl red indicator: Dissolve 0.1g methyl red indicator in 60 ml ethanol and add distilled water to make the volume 100 ml.

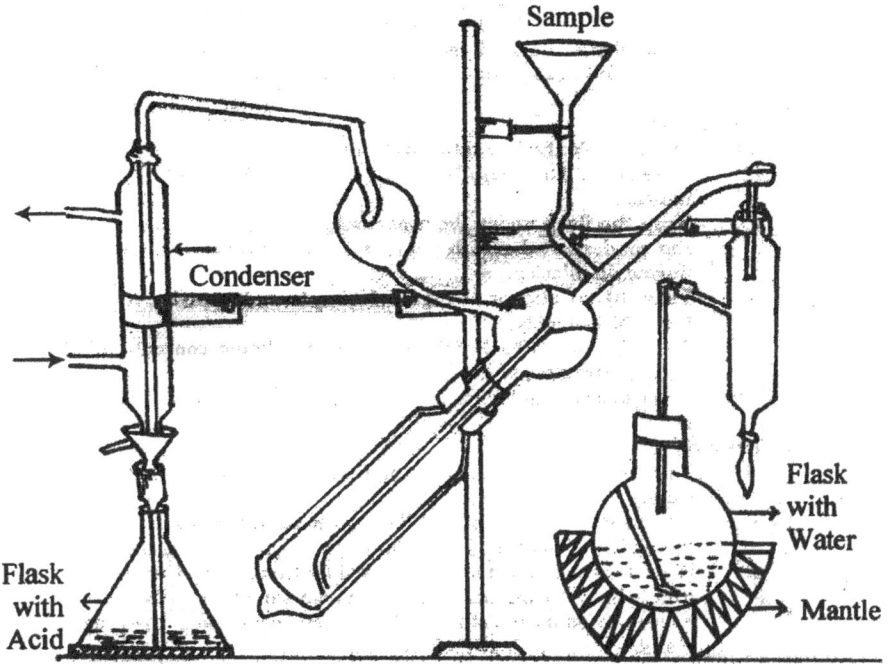

Fig.2: Micro Kjeldahl Distillation Assembly

Procedure
1. Digestion
i) Take 5 ml strained rumen liquor in a kjeldahl flask
ii) Add 10 ml concentrated H_2SO_4.
iii) Add 2-3 g digestion mixture.
iv) Keep the flask on digestion bench and allow gentle boiling. Bumping should be avoided.
v) When the solution becomes clear blue, then remove the flask from the digestion bench and cool it.
vi) Add 5 to 10 ml distilled water to the kjeldahl flask. Transfer the whole material in 100 ml volumetric flask with repeated washings of distilled water. Make the volume to 100 ml.

2. Distillation
i) Set the kjeldahl distillation assembly
ii) Take 10 ml 0.01N H_2SO_4 (A) in a conical flask and add 2-3 drops of indicator.
iii) Keep the flask under the condenser in such a way that the tip of the condenser should be dipped in acid, to avoid ammonia loss during distillation.
iv) Take 10 ml aliquot of digested sample and transfer it into the kjeldahl assembly.

v) Add 15-20 ml 40% NaOH to make the aliquot contents alkaline and put the stopper immediately.
vi) Allow distillation for 15 min.

3.   Titration
i) Remove the flask after washing tip of the condenser with distilled water.
ii) Titrate the contents of the flask with standard 0.01 N NaOH till the pink color develops (end point).
iii) Record the volume of alkali (B) used for titration on the burette.
iv) Run a blank using all reagents but no sample and following the whole procedure to estimate the nitrogen contents of the reagents, if any.

Calculation

1ml 0.01N H_2SO_4 = 0.00014 g nitrogen

$$\text{Nitrogen / 100ml rumen liquor} = \frac{V \times 0.00014 \times D \times 100}{v \times A} \times 100$$

Where, V = A — B
D = Dilution (Volume made in volumetric flask)
v = Initial volume of rumen liquor taken for the digestion
A = Aliquot taken (10 ml)

Total nitrogen of sample = Total nitrogen of sample - Total nitrogen of blank

Precaution

1. Bumping should not be allowed during digestion. Beads can be used to avoid bumping.
2. During distillation, first flask containing acid should be arranged under the condenser of the distillation assembly and thereafter alkali should be added in the sample. Because addition of alkali releases ammonia immediately.
3. Sample should be digested completely and clear blue color is the indication of complete digestion.

TCA Precipitable Nitrogen

TCA precipitable nitrogen is the nitrogen coming from the true protein because by adding trichloroacetic acid, only proteins are precipitated.

Rumen Liquor Analysis

These precipitated proteins are analyzed further for nitrogen contents by microkjeldahl method as described above.

Procedure
1. Take 5.0 ml rumen liquor in a centrifuge tube.
2. Add 5.0 ml of 20% TCA
3. Leave the tubes overnight.
4. Centrifuge the tubes at 2,000 rpm for 10 min.
5. Transfer the whole precipitate with repeated washings of distilled water in kjeldahl flask.
6. Proceed for digestion, distillation and titration as described above.

Soluble Nitrogen
TCA precipitable nitrogen subtracted from total nitrogen gives soluble nitrogen contents of rumen liquor.

Ammonia Nitrogen
In alkaline medium, ammonia is released from the rumen liquor and the released ammonia is analyzed for nitrogen contents by micro-kjeldahl method.

Procedure
1. Take 5.0 ml strained rumen liquor in the distillation assembly and 5 ml of 40% NaOH.
2. Proceed for distillation and titration as described above.

Lactic Acid
Lactic acid, when heated with concentrated H_2SO_4, converts into acetaldehyde, which reacts with p-hydroxydiphenyl to give purple color in the presence of copper ions (Barker and Summerson, 1941).

Reagents
1. Copper sulphate 20% : Dissolve 200g $CuSO_4\ 5H_2O$ in 500 ml distilled water and make the volume to one litre. The solution is stable indefinitely.
2. Copper sulphate 4% : Take 200 ml of reagent 1. and make the volume to one litre.
3. Calcium hydroxide $(Ca(OH)_2)$.
4. Concentrated H_2SO_4.
5. NaOH 5% - 5g NaOH, dissolve in 100 ml distilled water.
6. p-hydroxydiphenyl reagent : Take 1.5 g p-hydroxydiphenyl in a log ml volumetric flask. Add 10 ml of 5% NaOH and 10 ml distilled water. Warm it with constant stirring to dissolve. Make the volume to 100 ml. Store it in amber color bottle.

7. Stock standard lactic acid : Take 0.1065g lithium lactate in 100 ml volumetric flask and dissolve in about 50 ml distilled water. Add 0.1 ml concentrated H_2SO_4 and make up the volume to 100 ml with distilled water. The solution contains 1 mg lactic acid per ml and the solution is stable for a long period in refrigerator.
8. Working standard lactic acid solution: Dilute 1 ml of stock lactic acid solution to 100 ml with distilled water. It contains 0.01 mg lactic acid per ml. Prepare fresh working solution at the time of analysis.

Procedure
1. Take 1 ml strained rumen liquor in a centrifuge tube. Add 1 ml of 20% $CuSO_4$ and make the volume to 10 ml.
2. Add 1g $Ca(OH)_2$, shake vigorously to make the mixture homogenous.
3. Leave the tubes for 90 minutes with periodic shaking.
4. Centrifuge at 3000 rpm for 10 min.
5. Take 1 ml supernatant in a test tube in duplicate.
6. Add 0.05 ml of 4% $CuSO_4$.
7. Add 6 ml concentrated H_2SO_4 drop by drop with continuous shaking.
8. Keep the tubes in boiling water bath for 5 minutes.
9. Cool the tubes at room temperature.
10. Add 0.1 ml p-hydroxydiphenyl reagent drop by drop. The pipette tip should not touch the wall of the tube. Mix the contents immediately and vigorously.
11. Incubate the tubes at 30°C for 30 min with periodic shaking.
12. Keep the tubes in boiling water bath for 90sec. Remove the tubes and cool to room temperature.
13. To plot the standard curve prepare the standard tubes in duplicate as follows:

Tube No.	1	2	3	4	5	6
Distilled water (ml)	1.00	0.9	0.8	0.6	0.4	0.2
Standard lactic acid solution (ml)	0.0	0.1	0.2	0.4	0.6	0.8
Lactic acid concentration (µg)	0.0	1.0	2.0	4.0	6.0	8.0

14. Proceed for color development (step 5 to 12).
15. Read absorbance (optical density) of all the tubes at 560nm.
16. Find out the concentration of sample on standard curve and multiply by 10 (dilution) to give µg lactic acid/ml rumen liquor.

(B) Rumen Microbial Enzymes

Handling of Enzymes
Enzymes are very fragile substances and very soon undergo denaturation and inactivation under unsuitable conditions. Precautions should be taken

to protect the enzymes from inactivation during handling them. Although the suitable conditions vary with different enzymes but there are a few points which are applicable to most of the enzymes.

Temperature
High temperatures are always detrimental for the enzymes. Care should be taken not to expose the enzymes above body temperature, even at body temperature not for a longer time. During the process of isolation and purification a temperature of about 4°C should be maintained.

pH
Highly acidic and alkaline conditions are destructive for the enzymes. In general, majority of enzymes are inactivated below pH 5.0 and above pH 9.0, though exceptions are there. Thus while adjusting pH by adding acid or alkali, the drop should go slowly down the side of the vessel, with gentle and continuous stirring of the solution to avoid. formation of destruction zones around the drops. It is always preferred to maintain pH at neutral during handling the enzymes

Froth Formation
Enzyme preparation should be transferred very carefully to avoid frothing because many enzymes denature at the surface. Thus the enzyme solution should be poured by the side of the vessel to avoid entry of air bubbles.

Organic Solvents
Organic solvents like alcohol, acetone etc. inactivate the enzymes. Use of organic solvents should be avoided but if requried, precaution should be taken while adding it and should be added at low temperature (-15 to -20°C) and very slowly with continuous and gentle stirring.

Detergents
Use of detergents should be avoided as they also inactivate the enzymes. Especially anionic detergents like sodium dodecyl sulphate (SDS), sodium deoxycholate (DOC) or cationic detergents like cetyltrimethylammonium bromide (CTAB) etc. should not be used. Some times a nonionic detergent like triton x 100 is used for breaking the cells to release the enzymes. It should be used at a very low concentration with short treatment time.

Storage
The enzymes should be stored in deep-freeze where they are stable even for a few months. Repeated freezing-thawing should be avoided because it results in loss of activity. Sometimes enzymes can be stored in a precipitated form in saturated ammonium sulfate solution. When required,

they can be centrifuged down and dissolved in water. It is always recommended to store the enzyme preparation in small aliquots for one time use. Enzymes in concentrated form are more stable than in diluted form.

Bacterial Contamination
Enzyme preparations should be protected from bacterial contamination while storing for a long period by adding protectants like sodium azide etc.

Practical Precautions During Enzyme Estimation
While estimating the enzyme activity, to maintain linearity of the reaction, the conditions in the reaction mixture must be maintained as constant as possible.

Temperature
Reaction should be carried out in thermostatic conditions. All the reagents to be used for the reaction must be brought at a required temperature before mixing them to start the reaction. For each enzyme the optimum temperature for its maximum activity is different, so the enzyme reaction should be carried out at optimum temperature for the enzyme, to get maximum activity. If not possible then carryout the enzyme reaction at ambient temperature.

Buffering System
Activity of an enzyme is maximum at a particular pH called optimium pH for that particular enzyme and little change in the pH, changes its rate of reaction. Therefore when an enzyme activity is estimated, a recommended pH should be maintained throughout the reaction, and for that proper buffereing system has to be provided for the asssay mixture to prevent the change in pH during the reaction.

Contamination
Enzymes are highly catalytic in nature so any contamination in the vessel should be avoided which can stimulate or inhibit the reaction. eg . in case of amylase estimation, slight contamination of saliva during pipetting in the reaction mixture will increase the enzyme activity many folds. Thus pipetting should be done very carefully and glassware should be washed properly.

Reaction Rate
Reaction rate should not be very fast or slow and should be adjusted in such a way that the readings could be made properly and with in the range. The reaction rate can be adjusted by increasing or decreasing the volume

of the enzyme in the reaction mixture. Care should be taken that enzyme volume should not be very large in assay mixture. It is preferable to have enzyme preparation in the concentrated form so that very small quantity of the enzyme sample may be sufficient to get reaction within the range.

Mixing
When the reaction is started either by adding substrate or enzyme in the assay mixture, immediate thorough mixing is required because reaction starts immediately as soon as substrate and enzyme come in contact with each other.

Apparatus
1. Ice machine
2. Refrigerated centrifuge
3. Spectrophotometer
4. Sonicator
5. Deep fridge
6. pH meter
7. Balance
8. Magnetic stirrer with magnets
9. Ice box
10. Pipettes
11. Beakers
12. Measuring cylinders
13. Volumetric flasks
13. Storage tubes
14. Test tubes

Fractionation of Rumen Liquor for Enzyme Estimation

Reagents
1. Phosphate buffer 0.1 M, pH 6.8
Solution 1: Dissolve 17.799 g $Na_2HPO_4.2H_2O$ to make the volume 1 litre.
Solution 2: Dissolve 15.601 $NaH_2PO_4.2H_2O$ to make the volume 1 litre.
Take solution 1. and adjust pH to 6.8 by adding solution 2.

Procedure
Rumen liquor is collected through a permanent fistula in the rumen or with the help of a stomach tube. The frequency of rumen liquor collection may vary with the type of study and in most cases, it is at 4 h post feeding for enzyme estimation. The collection should be done at 39°C ± 2°C in a conical flask and plug it tightly. Transport the flask immediately to the laboratory for processing.

Protozoa Rich Fraction

Take 20 ml of thoroughly mixed SRL and centrifuge at 450 x g for 5 min at 37°C. Decant the supernatant and store it in a labeled test tube for further fractionation. The pellet formed in the centrifuge tube is suspended in the starting volume (20 ml) of 0.1 M phosphate buffer pH 7.0. Centrifuge again at 450 x g for 5 min at 4°C and remove the supernatant. Repeat the process twice and suspend the finally washed pellet in 10 ml of phosphate buffer.

Bacteria Rich Fraction

The supernatant collected after the removal of protozoa is centrifuged at 27000 x g at 37°C for 30 min. The entire supernatant is removed and used as cell-free rumen fluid. The bacterial pellet left in the centrifuge tube is washed thrice with phosphate buffer as in the case of protozoa but centrifugation is done each time at 27000 x g at 4°C for 30 min. The washed bacterial pellet is suspended in 10 ml phosphate buffer.

Disruption of Protozoa and Bacteria Rich Fractions

The protozoa and bacteria rich fractions kept in ice bath, are disrupted by sonication at 10µ for 5 min with 30 sec break. It is followed by centrifugation at 27000 x g for 30 min at 4°C. The supernatant of each fraction is used as the source of protozoal and bacterial enzymes.

Measure the volume of cell free fraction, protozoa rich fraction and bacteria rich fraction (A, B and C) and estimate the protein concentration.

Calculation for Converting 'g' into rpm (Revolutions Per Minute) for Centrifugation

$g = r \, (rpm)^2 \times 118 \times 10^{-7}$
Where, r = radius

Protein Estimation

Protein estimation by Lowry method (1951) is done by the formation of copper protein complex in the alkaline medium. This complex then reduces a phosphomolybdic-phosphotungstate reagent to yield intense blue color.

Reagents

1. Standard solution of bovine serum albumin (0.06% BSA): It is prepared in distilled water to contain 0.6 mg BSA/ml.
2. Trichloroacetic acid (TCA) 10% solution: Dissolve 10 g TCA in distilled water to make the volume 100 ml.

Rumen Liquor Analysis

3. Solution A; Dissolve 2 g sodium carbonate in 100 ml of 0.1N NaOH solution.
4. Solution B: Dissolve 1 g sodium-potassium tartrate in 100 ml distilled water. Add to it 0.5 g copper sulphate and keep it overnight and then filter to remove the precipitate, if any. Solution A and B can be stored at room temperature.
5. Solution C: Mix 50 ml solution A and 1 ml solution B just before the use.
6. Solution D: Mix 1 ml Folin and Ciocalteu's phenol reagent and 2 ml distilled water just before use.

Procedure
1. Take 0.1 ml sample and 0.4 ml distilled water in a test tube in duplicate.
2. Standard curve; Prepare tubes of standard BSA in duplicate as follows:

Tube No.	1	2	3	4	5	6	7	8	9	10	11
Standard BSA (ml)	0.0	0.05	0.10	0.15	0.20	0.25	0.30	0.35	0.40	0.45	0.50
Dist. Water (ml)	0.50	0.45	0.50	0.45	0.30	0.25	0.20	0.15	0.10	0.05	0.00
BSA (µg)	000	30	60	90	120	150	180	210	240	270	300

3. Add 5 ml solution C in all the tubes and leave for 10 min at room temperature.
4. Add 0.5 ml solution D and mix it immediately and vigorously.
5. After 10 min record absorbance (A) against blank at 600 nm.
6. Prepare calibration curve by plotting "A" against standard BSA solutions.
7. Calculate the protein concentration mg/ml by reading the absorbance of sample on standard curve.

Precautions
The Folins reagent is stable only in the acidic medium therefore while adding it in the alkaline copper protein complex it should be mixed immediately and thoroughly to get it reduced before it breaks down due to alkaline medium.

Expression of Enzyme Activity
The enzyme activities in the three fractions can be expressed in the following ways.

Fraction	Volume of the fraction (ml) V	Protein mg/ml (a)	Total protein (a x V = b)	Units/ml (c)	Specific activity (%$_a$ = d) a	Total units (b x d = e)	Units / 100 ml SRL (%$_{20}$) x 100
Cell free fraction							
Protozoa rich fraction							
Bacteria rich fraction							

* Starting volume of rumen liquor taken for the fractionation.

Fibre Degrading Enzymes

1. Carboxymethyl Cellulase (Endo-1, 4-β-glucanase, EC 3.2.1.4)

Principle

The enzyme catalyses the hydrolysis of cellulose, releasing glucose by breaking the (β-1, 4-linkages. The enzyme is of microbial origin. The amount of glucose released is measured colorimetrically to estimate the enzyme activity (Miller 1959; Agarwal *et al.*, 1990).

The enzyme is active against cellodextrins, phosphoric acid swollen cellulose, carboxymethyl cellulose and hydroxymethyl cellulose. Carboxymethyl cellulose is the most common substrate used for the estimation of enzyme activity.

Reagents
1. 0.1M phosphate buffer, pH 6.8.
2. Carboxymethyl cellulose (1%): Dissolve 1 g of carboxymethyl cellulose in distilled water and dilute to 100 ml.
3. Dinitrosalicylic acid (DNS) solution: Dissolve 10 g of sodium hydroxide pellets in 500 ml distilled water. Add 10 g DNS and 2g phenol and dilute to 1 litre with distilled water. Sodium sulphite (0.05%) is added just before use.
4. Rochelle salt solution (40%): Dissolve 40 g of Rochelle salt (sodiumpotassium tartrate) in distilled water and make volume to 100 ml.
5. Standard solution of glucose (0. 1%): Dissolve 10 mg of glucose in 10 ml distilled water.

Rumen Liquor Analysis

Procedure
1. (a) Test : Take 1.0 ml phosphate buffer, 0.5 ml sample and in a test tube and 0.5 ml carboxymethyl cellulose solution in a test tube and mix well. Incubate the tubes for 1h at 39°C. Stop the reaction by adding 3 ml DNS.
   (b) Control : Mix 1.0 ml phosphate buffer, 0.5 ml sample in a test tube. Add 3 ml DNS and then 0.5 ml carboxymehtyl cellulose solution.
   (c) Blank : 2 ml distilled water and 3 ml DNS reagent.
   (d) Standard : Prepare tubes in duplicate with the standard glucose solution and distilled water to plot a calibration curve as follows:

Tube No.	1	2	3	4	5	6	7	8	9
Distt. Water (ml)	2.00	1.75	1.50	1.25	1.00	0.75	0.5	0.25	0.00
St. Glucose Sol. (ml)	0.00	0.25	0.50	0.75	1.00	1.25	1.50	1.75	2.00
Glucose conc. (mg)	0.00	0.25	0.50	0.75	1.00	1.25	1.50	1.75	2.00

2. Add 3 ml DNS regent in all the tubes.
3. Keep all the tubes in boiling water bath for 10 min.
4. Add 1 ml. Rochelle salt solution in each tube and then cool them to room temperature.
5. Make up the volume to 20 ml with distilled water.
6. Read optical density (OD) at 575 nm against blank.
7. Prepare calibration curve by plotting OD against glucose concentration.

Calculations

Change in OD A = test - control

Read A on the calibration curve to get the µg glucose released.

$$\text{Enzyme activity Units/ml} = \mu\text{mol glucose /h/ml} = \frac{\mu g\ glucose}{T \times S \times 160}$$

Where,
T = time of incubation (1 h),
S = volume of sample (0.5 ml)
160 = molecular weight of glucose

Note : DNS solution can be stored at room temperature for a month in amber color bottle without adding sodium sulphite. Sodium sulphite should be added at the time of use.

2. α-Amylase (1,4- α-D-Glucanohydrolase, EC 3.2.1.1.)

Principle
The enzyme attacks on α-1,4-glucan linkages of starch and glycogen, releasing maltose, isomaltose, larger oligo-saccharides and glucose. The α-amylase activity is determined by measuring the rate of release of reducing sugars during the incubation of enzyme with the substrate.

Procedure
The procedure for estimation of a-amylase activity is similar to that of Endo-1, 4-α-glucanase with the following differences.
1. Starch solution (1%): Dissolve 1 g starch in 90 ml of distilled water by heating. Make up the volume to 100 ml.
2. Assay mixture : It contains 0.5 ml phosphate buffer, 0.25 ml starch solution and 0.25 ml sample.
3. Incubation time: 30 min.
4. Enzyme activity is expressed as gmol reducing sugars released per min per ml.

3. Xylanase (1,4-β-xylan xylano hydrolase; Endo-1,4-β-xylanase; EC 3.2.1.8)

Principle
The xylanase catalyses, hydrolysis of xylan and releases its structural unit D-xylose by breaking (β-1, 4 linkages. The enzyme is of microbial origin. The activity of the enzyme is determined by estimating colorimetrically the amount of D-xylose released during incubation of enzyme with substrate.

Procedure
The procedure for estimation of activity xylanase is similar to that of Endo-1, 4-α-glucanase with the following differences
1. 0.25% xylan solution: Dissolve 250 mg xylan (from oat spelt) in 100 ml distilled water.
2. Standard solution of D-xylose (0.1%): Dissolve 100 mg of xylose in 100 ml distilled water.
3. Assay mixture: 1 ml phosphate buffer, 0.5 ml sample and 0.5 ml xylan solution.
4. Incubation time: 30 min.
5. Standard curve: Prepare tubes as follows

Tube No	1	2	3	4	5	6
Dist. Water (ml)	2.0	1.7	1.4	1.1	0.8	0.5
Stand. Xylose Sol. (ml)	0.0	0.3	0.6	0.9	1.2	1.5
Xylose Conc. (µg)	000	300	600	900	1200	1500

6. Enzyme activity Units/ml = µmol xylose/min/ml = $\dfrac{\mu g \text{ xylose}}{T \times S \times 150}$

Where, 150 is the molecular weight of xylose

4. β-Glucosidase (β-D-Glucoside glucohydrolase, EC 3.2.1.21)

Principle
The enzyme catalyses the hydrolysis of cellobiose and short chain oligosaccharides to release glucose. β-glucosidase is active towards salicin, phosphoric acid swollen cellulose, cellobiose and p-nitrophenol β-D-glucopyranoside (PNPG).

With PNPG as a substrate, the enzyme activity is determined by measuring the amount of p-nitrophenol released during incubation of substrate with the enzyme (Shewale and Sadana, 1978).

Reagents
1. 0.1M phosphate buffer pH 6.8.
2. PNPG solution (0.1%): Dissolve 100 mg of PNPG in 100 ml phosphate'
    buffer. Store in amber color bottle in fridge.
3. p-nitrophenol solution (0.01%): Dissolve 10 mg of p-nitrophenol in 100 ml distilled water.
4. Sodium carbonate solution (2%): Dissolve 2 g of sodium carbonate in 100 ml distilled water.

Procedure
1. (a) Test : Mix 0.1 ml. enzyme and 0.9 ml. PNPG solution. Incubate the tubes for 10 min at 39°C. Stop the reaction by adding 1 ml sodium carbonate.
    (b) Control: Mix 0.1 ml enzyme and 1 ml sodium carbonate. Then add 0.9 ml PNPG solution.
    (c) Blank : 1 ml distilled water and 1 ml sodium carbonate.

(e) Standard : Prepare tubes of graded concentration of p-nitrophenol in duplicate to plot calibration curve as follows

Tube No.	1	2	3	4	5	6	7	8
Dist. Water (ml)	1.000	0.98	0.96	0.94	0.92	0.90	0.85	0.80
p-nitrophenol (ml)	0.000	0.02	0.04	0.06	0.08	0.10	0.15	0.20
p-nitrophenol (ug)	0.0	2.0	4.0	6.0	8.0	10.0	15.0	20.0

2. Add 1 ml sodium carbonate solution to the standard tubes.
3. Read optical density (OD) at 400 nm against blank.
4. Prepare a calibration curve by plotting OD against standard p-nitrophenol concentration.

Calculations

Change in absorbance A for sample = test - control
Read A on calibration curve to get the amount (µg) of p- nitrophenol released.

$$\text{Enzyme activity (Units)} = \mu\text{mol p-nitrophenol/min/ml} = \frac{\mu g\ p\text{ - nitrophenol}}{T \times S \times 139.11}$$

Where, T= 10 min and S= 0. 1 ml, 139. 11 = molecular weight of p-nitrophenol

5. α-Glucosidase (EC 3.2.1.21)

Principle
α-Glucosidase is an enzyme which breaks linkages of disacchafides releasing its structural units. The enzyme group includes sucrase (sucrose D-glucohydrolase, EC 2.2.1.20), isomaltase (dextrin, D-glucanohydrolase, EC 3.2.1.10).

The enzyme activity is determined by measuring the amount of p- nitrophenol released during the incubation of the enzyme with the substrate p-nitrophenyl α-D glucopyranoside.

Procedure
Procedure for α-glucosidase estimation is same as for β-glucosidase with the only difference that here the substrate is 0.1% p-nitrophenyl-α-D-glucopyranoside.

6. β-Xylosidase (1,4-α-D-xylan xylohydrolase: Exo-1, 4-β-D xylosidase, EC 3.2.1.37)

Principle
Hemicellulose is predominantly the xylo-glucan polymers in plant tissue which on hydrolysis releases small chain xylose polymers and xylose. β-xylosidase further hydrolyses these small polymers to release xylose.

Using p-nitrophenyl β-D xylopyranoside as a substrate, the activity of the enzyme is determined colorimetrically by measuring the amount of p-nitrophenol released during incubation of the enzyme with the substrate.

Procedure
Procedure for β-xylosidase estimation is similar as that for β-glucosidase with the only difference that here the substrate is 0.1% p-nitrophenyl-β-D-xylopyranoside.

Protein and NPN Degrading Enzymes

1. Urease (Urea Amidohydrolase, EC 3.5.1.5)

Principle
Urease enzyme hydrolyses urea to generate ammonia. The enzyme activity is determined by measuring the amount of ammonia produced during the incubation of enzyme with urea (Weatherburn, 1967).

Reagents
1. 0.1 mM phosphate buffer, pH 6.8.
2. 10 mM urea solution: Dissolve 15 mg urea and 8 mg EDTA disodium salt in 25 ml phosphate buffer.
3. Solution A: Dissolve 1 g phenol in 50 ml distilled water. Add 5 mg sodium nitroprusside, dissolve and make the volume to 100 ml with distilled water.
4. Solution B: Dissolve 0.5 g NaOH in 50 ml distilled water. Add 0.84 ml sodium hypochlorite and make the volume to 100 ml with distilled water. Solution A and B are to be stored in amber colour bottles in refrigerator.
5. Stock standard solution of ammonium sulphate: Dissolve 0.048 g ammonium sulphate in 100 ml distilled water to get a final concentration of 10 mg of ammonia nitrogen per 100 ml of solution.
6. Working standard: Standard solution of ammonium sulphate: Take 10 ml solution 5 and make up to 100 ml. The solution contain 0.01 mg ammonia nitrogen per ml.

Procedure

1. (a) **Test** : Take 0.5 ml buffer, 0.25 ml sample and 0.25 ml urea solution in a test tube. Incubate the tube for 15 min at 39°C. Add 5 ml solution A and mix vigorously.
   (b) **Control** : Take 0.5 ml buffer and 0.25 ml sample. First add to it Solution A then 0.25 ml urea solution.
   (c) **Blank** : 1 ml distilled water, solution A.
   (d) **Standard** : Prepare tubes of graded concentration of ammonia nitrogen (ammonium sulphate solution) in duplicate for plotting a calibration curve as follows:

Tube No.	1	2	3	4	5	6	7	8
Dist. Water (ml)	1.00	0.95	0.90	0.80	0.60	0.40	0.20	0.00
Standard Sol. (ml)	0.00	0.05	0.10	0.20	0.40	0.60	0.80	1.00
Ammonium nitrogen (µg)	0.00	0.5	1.0	2.0	4.0	6.0	8.0	1.0

2. Add 5 ml solution A in the standard tubes.
3. Immediately after adding solution A add solution B in all the tubes, mix the contents vigorously.
4. Incubate all the tubes for 15 min at 39°C for colour development.
5. Record optical density (OD) at 625 nm against blank.
6. Prepare calibration curve by plotting OD against standard ammonia nitrogen concentration.

Calculations

Change in absorbance A for sample = test- control
Read A on calibration curve to get the amount (µg) of ammonia nitrogen released.
Enzyme activity (Units) = µmol ammonia nitrogen/min/ml =

$$\frac{\mu g \text{ ammonia nitrogen}}{T \times S \times 14}$$

Where,
T = 10 min and S = 0.1 ml, 14 = molecular weight of nitrogen

2. Proteases

Principle

Feed proteins are hydrolysed successively into peptides and amino acids by the action of proteolytic enzymes. The enzymes proteases are present both in animal tissues and in microorganisms.

Rumen Liquor Analysis

The activity of these enzymes is determined by measuring the amount of proteins hydrolysed during incubation of the substrate with the enzyme.

Reagents
1. 0.1M phosphate buffer, pH 6.8.
2. Casein solution (1%): Dissolve 1 g casein in minimum volume of I N NaOH. Adjust pH 7.5 by adding 1 N HCl and make the final volume 100 ml with phosphate buffer.
3. Reagents for protein estimation (Lowry method)

Procedure
1. Test : Take 1.5 ml buffer, 0.25 ml casein solution and 0.25 ml sample in a test tube and incubate for 2 h at 39°C and then stop reaction by adding 2 ml. TCA soln.
2. Control : Mix 1.5 ml buffer, 0.25 ml sample and 2 ml TCA. After adding TCA, add 0.25 ml casein solution.
3. Keep the tubes overnight.
4. Next day centrifuge at 2500 rpm for 10 min and collect the supernatant.
5. Take 0.5 ml of the supernatant in a test tube for protein estimation

Calculation
Change in OD "A" = test - control
Read A on the calibration curve to get the µg hydrolyzed protein released.
Enzyme activity (Units) = µg hydrolyzed protein /min/ml = $\dfrac{\mu g \text{ hydrolyzed protein}}{T \times S}$

Transaminases

3. Aspartate Aminotransaminase : Glutamic Oxaloacetic Transaminase; GOT (EC 2.6.1.1.)

4. Alanine Aminotransaminase : Glutamic Pyruvic Transaminase; GPT (EC 2.6.1.2)

The enzymes, GOT and GPT catalyses the following reactions.

$$\text{Glutamic acid + oxaloacetic acid} \xleftrightarrow{\text{GOT}} \alpha\text{-ketoglutaric acid + Aspartic acid}$$

$$\text{Glutamic Acid + Pyruvic acid} \xleftrightarrow{\text{GPT}} \alpha\text{-ketoglutaric acid + Alanine}$$

The reactions are reversible. Colorimetric estimation of the enzyme activity is done in backward reaction. GPT activity is determined by measuring the amount of pyruvic acid released during incubation of the substrate with the enzyme. Pyruvic acid gives brown colour of hydrazone, formed by its reaction with 2,4-dinitrophenyl hydrazine (DNPH). In GOT, oxaloacetic acid is released during incubation of the substrate and the enzyme converts it spontaneously into pyruvic acid by decarboxylation. The pyruvic acid thus finally is estimated for measuring GOT acitivity (Reitman and Frankel, 1957).

Reagents
1. 0.1mM phosphate buffer, pH 7.4.
2. GOT substrate: Dissolve 2.66 g DL-aspartic acid in a minimum volume of 1N NaOH. Adjust pH to 7.4 and add 0.028 g α-ketoglutaric acid. Dissolve it by adding little more 1 N NaOH. Adjust pH to 7.4 and make it to 100 ml with phosphate buffer. Store it frozen in small aliquots of 10 ml.
3. GPT substrate : Dissolve 1.8 g alanine in water and adjust pH to 7.4 by additing 1 N NaOH, add 0.028 g α-ketoglutaric acid and dissolve it by adding a little more 1 N NaOH. Adjust pH to 7.4 and make it 100 ml with phosphate buffer. Store it frozen in small aliquots of 10 ml.
4. 4mM pyruvate standard: Dissolve 11 mg sodium pyruvate in 25 ml phosphate buffer. Store frozen in 1 ml aliquots.
5. 1m M 2,4-dinitrophenylhydrazine (DNPH): Dissolve 18.8 mg DNPH in 10 ml of concentrated hydrochloric acid and make upto 100 ml with distilled water. Store in brown bottle at room temperature.
6. 0.4N Sodium hydroxide: Dissolve 16 g NaOH in distilled water and make upto 1 litre.

Procedure (GOT)
1. (a) Test : Take 0. 1 ml sample and 0.5 ml substrate in a tube and incubate for 60 min at 39°C.
   (b) Control : Take 0.1 ml sample and 0.5 ml substrate. No incubation is required.
   (c) Pyruvate standard: Take 0.4 ml substrate, 0. 1 ml pyruvate solution and 0. 1 ml distilled water. No incubation is required.
   (d) Blank : 0. 5 ml substrate and 0. 1 ml distilled water.
2. Add 0.5 ml DNPH immediately and leave the tubes for 20 min at room temperature.
3. Add 5 ml of 0.4N sodium hydroxide.
4. Record optical density (OD) at 510 nm against reagent blank.

Rumen Liquor Analysis

Calculations
Enzyme activity is expressed as gmol pyruvate produced per litre sample per min =

$$\frac{T-C}{S-B} \times \frac{0.4 \times 1}{60} \times \frac{1000}{0.1} = \frac{T-C}{S-B} \times 67\mu mol$$

Procedure (GPT)
The procedure for GPT estimation is same as for GOT with the following differences.
1. Use GPT substrate
2. Incubation time for (a) test is 30 min.
3. Enzyme activity.

μmol pyruvate produced per litie sample per min =

$$\frac{T-C}{S-B} \times \frac{0.4 \times 1}{60} \times \frac{1000}{0.1} = \frac{T-C}{S-B} \times 133\mu mol$$

Conversion of μmol Pyruvvate/min/litre in to International Units (IU)

Calculated pyruvate (μmol/min/ml)	IU GOT	IU GPT
2	2	1
4	3	2
6	5	2
8	6	3
10	7	4
12	9	4
14	11	5
16	13	6
18	15	7
20	17	7
22	19	8
24	21	9
26	23	9
28	25	10
30	27	11
32	29	12
34	31	13
36	33	14
38	35	15

Contd...

40	37	16
42	39	17
44	41	18
46	44	19
48	47	20
50	51	21
52	55	22
54	60	23
56	-	24
58	-	25
60	-	26
62	-	27
64	-	29
66	-	30
68	-	31
70	-	33
72	-	34
74	-	35
76	-	36
78	-	37
80	-	38
82	-	39
84	-	40
86	-	42
88	-	44
90	-	46
92	-	48
94	-	50
96	-	52
98	-	54
100	-	56
102	-	60

5. Glutamate Dehydrogenase (GDH) (L-Glutamate : NAD$^+$ oxidoreductase E-C 1.4.1.2 and L-Glutamate : NADP$^+$ oxidoreductase EC 1.4.1.4)

The microorganisms utilize GDH pathway for ammonia assimilation to convert α-ketoglutaric acid into glutamic acid. The enzyme catalyzes the reaction.

$$NH_4^+ + \alpha\text{-ketoglutarate} + NADPH \longleftrightarrow glutamate + NADP^+ + H_2O$$
$$\text{or}$$
$$NH_4^+ + \alpha\text{-ketoglutarate} + NADH \longleftrightarrow glutamate + NAD^+ + H_2O$$

Rumen Liquor Analysis

GDH activity is determined by measuring the rate of change in absorbance
at 340 nm, due to oxidation of NADPH to $NADP^+$ and NADH to NAD^+
(Wolf and Wiliams, 1973; Bergmeyer, 1974).

Reagents
1. 0.075M Tris-HCl buffer: Dissolve 0.908g Tris in distilled water. Adjust pH 7.8 with HCl and make volume upto 100 ml.
2. 0.15M α-ketoglutarate: Dissolve 0.218g α-ketoglptarate in distilled water, adjust pH to 7.8 and make up the volume to 10ml.
3. 7.5mM reduced Nicotinamide-adenine-dinucleotide phosphate (NADPH): Dissolve 0.029g NADPH in 5ml distilled water.
4. 1.2 M Ammonium chloride: Dissolve 0.64 NH_4Cl in 10 ml distilled water.

Procedure
1. Prepare Blank and Test for each sample directly in the cuvette.
2. To both the tubes, take 1.0 ml buffer, 0.05 ml NH_4Cl, 0.1 ml sample and 0.05 ml NADPH. Add 0.3 ml distilled water in "Blank" and 0.2 ml in "Test".
3. Incubate the tubes at room temperature for 10 min.
4. Read the optical density (E_1) of Blank. Take another reading after 5 min. (E_2).
5. To the "Test" tube add O.1ml α-ketoglutaric acid and read the optical density (E_3) take another reading after 5 min (E_4).

Calculations
1. $E_1 - E_2 = A$
2. $E_3 - E_4 = B$
3. Change in optical density "A" / 5 minutes = B-A

$$\text{IU/liter or mU/ml} = \frac{A \times V}{e \times d \times v \times t} \times 10^6$$

Where,
e = Molar extinction coefficient of NADPH at 340 nm = 6.22 x 10^3 Liters/mole x cm.
d = diameter of the cuvette in cm = 1 cm
V = Total volume = 1.5 ml
v = Sample volume = O. 10 ml
T = Time = 5 minutes

6. Glutamate Synthase

The enzyme catalyses the reaction

$$\alpha\text{-ketoglutarate} + \text{L-glutamine} + \text{NADPH} \longrightarrow 2\text{L-glutamate} + \text{NADP}^+$$

or

$$\alpha\text{-Ketoglutarate} + \text{L-glutamine} + \text{NADH} \longrightarrow 2\text{ L-glutamate} + \text{NAD}^+$$

Both NADPH specific (EC 1.4.1.14) and NADH specific (EC 1.4.1.13) are present in microbes but the former is more active.

The enzyme activity is estimated by measuring the rate of change in absorbance at 340 nm due to oxidation of NADPH or NADH (Meers *et al.*, 1970).

Reagents
1. HEPES buffer 0.1M pH 7.5: Dissolve 2.383g HEPES in 50 ml. distilled water. Adjust pH to 7.5 and make the volume to 100 ml.
2. Nicotinamide adenine dinucleotide phosphate reduced (NADPH). 2mM: Dissolve 0.0153g NADPH in 10 mi distilled water.
3. α-ketoglutaric acid 10mM: Dissolve 0.0146g α-ketoglutaric acid in distilled water. Adjust pH to 7.5 and make volume upto 10 ml.
4. L-glutamine 20 mM: Dissolve 0.029g L-glutamine in distilled water and make upto 10 ml.
5. Ethylenediaminetetra acetic acid, disodium salt dihydrate (EDTA): 0.1M: Dissolve 0.372 g EDTA in 10 ml buffer.

Procedure
1. Prepare blank and test directly in the cuvette.
2. To the both tubes, take 1.0 ml. HEPES buffer, 0.2 ml NADPH, 0.2 ml α-ketoglutaric acid, 0.2 ml EDTA and 0.2 ml. sample. Add to it 0.2 ml distilled water in blank.
3. Incubate the tubes at room temperature for 10 min.
4. Read the optical density (E_1) of Blank. Take another reading after 5 min. (E_2).
5. To the "Test" tube add 0.2ml L-glutamine and read the optical density (E_3) take another reading after 5 min (E_4) Enzyme activity is linear for about ½ minute.

Calculations
1. $E_1 - E_2 = A$
2. $E_3 - E_4 = B$

Change in optical density "A" / 3 minutes = B - A

$$\text{IU/liter or mU/ml} = \frac{A \times V}{e \times d \times v \times t} \times 10^6$$

Where,
e = Molar extinction coefficient of NADPH at 340 nm = 6.22×10^3 Liters/mole x cm.
d = diameter of the cuvette in cm = 1 cm
V = Total volume = 1.5 ml
v = Sample volume = 0.10 ml
T = Time = 5 minutes

7. Glutamine Synthetase (L-Glutamate: Ammonia Ligase) (E.C. 6.3.1.2)

The enzyme catalyses the biosynthesis of glutamine

$$\text{Glutamate + ammonia + ATP} \xrightleftharpoons[Mn^{2+}]{Mg^{2+}} \text{glutamine + ADP + Pi}$$

First of all the enzyme was studied in animal tissue but later on it was reported in microbes like *Lactobacillus arabinosus, Escherichia coli* etc. The presence of this enzyme is well established in rumen microbes.

Principle
The enzyme activity can be estimated by measuring the rate of formation of inorganic phosphate by following the method of Fiske and Subbarow. But when in the reaction, ammonia is replaced by hydroxylamine, the product released is Y-glutamylhydroxamate, which gives a characteristic brown colour on addition of $FeCl_3$. This is the principle of estimation of glutamine synthetase described here (Bender *et al.*, 1977).

Reagents
1. Imidozole-hydrochloride 1 M pH 7.15: Dissolve 10.454g imidazolehydrochloride in distilled water. Adjust pH 7.15 with KOH and make up to 100 ml.
2. Hydroxylamine-hydrochloride 0.8M: 0.556 g hydroxylamine hydrochloride in 10 ml distilled water.
3. Magnesium chloride 3M: Dissolve 2.85 magnesium chloride in 10 ml distilled water.
4. Monosodium glutamate 0.85 M: Dissolve 1.44g monosodium glutamate in 10 ml distilled water.
5. Adinosine triphosphate sodium salt 0.2M: Dissolve 1:102g ATP in 10 ml distilled water.
6. Stop mixture: Prepare stop mixture by maxing 55g of $FeCl_3 \cdot 6H_2O$, 20g of trichloro-acetic acid and 21 ml of concentrated HCl per liter.

Procedure
1. Prepare fresh stock assay mixture daily as follows:

Stock Soln.	Volume	Final concentration (mM)
Water	9.2	-
0.1M imidazole-hydrochloride	2.0	94
0.80M hydroxylamine hydrochloride	1.25	47
3.0M $MgCl_2$	0.4	56
0.85M monosodium glutamate	4.2	168

   Adjust pH of stock assay mixture with 10M KOH to pH 7.7 at room temperature.
2. Take 0.40 ml of stock assay mixture and add to it enzyme to make it 0.44 ml.
3. After 5 min of equilibration at 37°C, initiate the reaction by adding 0.06 ml of ATP soln.
4. Incubate it for 15 min. at 37°C.
5. Stop the reaction by adding 1.0 ml of "stop mixture" and vortex the tubes immediately to dissolve the precipitate that forms upon the addition of stop mixture".
6. Centrifuge the assay mixture and collect the clear supernatant.
7. Measure the absorbance of supernatant at 540 nm against blank.
8. Prepare blank by excluding ATP.

Calculations
Under these conditions 1 μmol of glutamyl hydroxamate gives 0.532 units of absorbance at 540 nm. One unit of glutamine synthetase is defined as the amount of enzyme producing 1μmol of glutamyl hydroxamate.

Chapter 8

ESTIMATION OF RUMEN MICROBIAL PROTEIN PRODUCTION FROM PURINE DERIVATIVES IN URINE

Principle

Nucleic acids leaving the rumen are mainly of microbial origin which are extensively digested in the small intestine and the purines liberated are absorbed. Only a small amount of absorbed purines are utilized by the host animal, the rest are metabolised forming hypoxanthine, xanthine, uric acid and allantoin. These metabolites are excreted mainly through urine. Therefore, with the understanding of how urinary excretion of purine derivatives (PD) respond to purine absorption i.e. the response curve of PD excretion to purine input into intestines, the microbial purine outflow from the rumen and the microbial N supply to the ruminant animal can be estimated by measuring the purine derivatives excretion through urine.

Sample Collection
a) Collect all the urine produced by the animal without mixing of faeces.
b) Urine collection should be made for more than 5 days to reduce the error due to the end of collection variation in urine output.
c) Collection can be made as a bulk for the whole period.
d) Urine is collected into a container with approximately 100 ml. of 10% H_2SO_4
e) Record the original weight of the urine. The daily urine output may be 0.5-2 lit in sheep and 20-30 lit. in cattle. Add tap water to constant weight (4Kg for sheep, 50 kg or more for cattle). So the final volume of diluted urine is the same for all animals and every day.

f) Mix the diluted urine thoroughly, filter some urine through glass wool or surgical gauze, take a subsample of 20 ml and store it at — 20°C.

Determination of Purine Derivatives

Dilution of Urine Samples
The urine samples which have been previously diluted before storage still needs further dilution. The next dilution should be to such an extent that the concentrations in the final samples will be with in the range of the standards used in the assays (5-50 mg/lit for both uric acid and allantoin).

Determination of Allantoin by Colorimetric Method

Principle
Allantoin is first hydrolysed under a weak alkaline condition at 100°C, to allantoic acid which is further degraded to urea and glyoxylic acid in weak acid solution. The glyoxylic acid then reacts with phenylhydrazine hydrochloride to produce a phenylhydrazone of the acid. The product then forms an unstable chromosphore with potassium ferricyanide. The colour is read at 522 nm.

Preparation of Standards
(a) Prepare an allantoin stock solution of 100mg/lit. Weigh 50 mg of allantoin and transfer it into a volumetric flask. Dissolve in about 100 ml 0.01 M NaOH and make up the volume with distilled water.
(b) Prepare working concentrations of 10, 20, 30, 40, 50 and 60 mg/l.
(c) Store each working standards as small aliquots in the freezer.

Procedure
(a) Pipette 1 ml of sample, standard or distilled water (blank) into 15 ml tubes
(b) Add 5 ml of distilled water.
(c) Add 1 ml of 0.5M NaOH.
(d) Mix the contents of the tubes by Vortexing.
(e) Put the tubes in the boiling water bath for 7 min.
(f) Remove from the boiling water and cool the tubes in the cold water.
(g) Add to each tube 1 ml of HCl (0.5M). The pH after adding HCl must be in the range of 2-3.
(h) Add 1 ml of phenylhydrazine solution (0.023 M freshly prepared). Mix and transfer the tubes again to the boiling water bath for exactly 7 min.
(i) Remove from the boiling water and dump it immediately into the icy alcohol bath for several minutes.

(j) Pipette 3 ml of conc. HCl (11.4N) (operate in a fume cupboard) and 1 ml of Potassium ferricyanide (0.05 M). Prepare K-ferricyanide freshly on the day of testing. Perform this for all samples within a shortest possible span. Start the timer.
(k) Mix thoroughly and transfer some to 4.5 ml cuvettes at room temperature.
(l) Read the absorbance at 522 nm after exactly 20 min. Once started, do it as quickly as possible.

Calculation
The standard curve is linear. Therefore, we can fit a linear regression between the known allantoin concentrations (Standards) (X) and the corresponding OD (Y). The slope of the line is usually 0.16-0.18. Calculate the concentration of the unknown based on thiS equation.

Determination of Allantoin by HPLC

Reagents
a) 1.0 g/L 2,4-dinitrophenylhydrazine (DNPH) dissolved in 2M HCl and filtered through Whatman No. 1 paper. Store at 4°C.
b) 0.6M NaOH
c) pH indicator: 0.04 (w/v) thymol blue, dissolved in distilled deionized water and filtered through Whatman No. 1 paper.
d) Allantoin standards: 5, 10, 20, 30, 40, 50 mg/l water.

Derivatization Procedure
a) Do a set of standard for each batch of derivatization.
b) Pipette 500 µl of a sample or standard to a 1.5 ml microcentrifuge tube.
c) Add 50 µl of the pH indicator. The colour of the mixture would be either yellow or red (red when pH<1.2).
d) Add 100µl of 0.6M NaOH solution.
e) Mix and observe the colour. If the colour fails to change to blue (pH>9.2 when blue), add 50 µl NaOH (volume to be recorded).
f) Repeat (e) if necessary
g) Cap tubes, mix. Place them in water bath at 85°C for 1 hour.
h) Transfer the tubes from the water bath, add 200µl of the DNPH solution. Mix. the colour of the mixture that would be orange-yellow.
i) Place the tubes back into the water bath to continue heating for another 20 min.
j) If the samples are not used for injection into HPLC right away, store the sample in the freezer.
k) Centrifuge the samples at 20,000 rpm for 25 min.

l) Carefully transfer 0.3 ml. or 0.5 ml of the supernatant into each sample vial.
m) Make sure that the vials are clearly labelled and there are no air bubbles in the vials.
n) These samples are now ready for injection. Store in the fridge if necessary.

Calculations
Calculate the concentrations of unknown with the known standards.

Determination of Xanthine Plus Hypoxanthine by Enzymatic Method
Principle

In this method, xanthine and hypoxanthine are enzymatically converted to uric acid and that uric acid is monitored by its absorbance at 293 nm. When the urine samples are treated with xanthine oxidase, xanthine and hypoxanthine are converted to uric acid. There should be an increase in OD at 293nm after the enzyme, treatment. The net increase is then used for the calculation of the amount of uric acid formed based on the uric acid standard curve.

Preparation of Standard
a) Prepare a stock uric acid solution of 100 mg/l. Dilute it to give working concentrations of 20, 40, 60, 80, 100mg/l.
b) Store each working standard as small quintities in the freezer.

Procedure
a) Pipette 1 ml of urine or standard or distilled water into a cuvette. All samples and standards are done in duplicates. Distilled water is used as the blank. Prepare two sets.
b) Add 2.5 ml phosphate buffer(KH_2PO_4 0.2 M, pH 7.35 adjust with either H_3PO_4 or KOH).
c) Add 0.35 ml of 4.3 mM-L-histidine solution and Mix.
d) In one set, add 250 µl of buffer, in the other set add 150 µl of the xanthine oxidase solution (xanthine oxidase 25 µl to 3 ml of the buffer).
e) Mix well and incubate at 37°C for 60 min.
f) Read OD at 293 nm.

Calculations
a) Use OD of the standards without XO added for construction of uric acid standard curve. Transform both X and Y into natural logarithmic function. Fit the Ln (Y) into a linear function of Ln (X).

b) Calculate the OD for the samples, i.e. the difference between two sets with and without XO addition: OD= OD with XO - OD without XO.
c) Calculate the corresponding concentration of uric acid from OD based on the above standard curve.
d) Estimate the contribution of OD reading from the xanthine (ODX) in the set without XO based on a predetermined xanthine standard curve.
e) Re-adjust the OD (i.e. OD_2 = OD + ODX) and repeat from step 3 once.
f) The uric acid standard curve is not linear, but when both X (concentration) and Y (OD) are transformed into Ln(X) and Ln (Y), LN (Y) becomes a linear function of Ln(X). This relationship is then used for the calculation of the concentrations of the samples from their OD readings.

Determination of Uric Acid by Uricase Method

Principle
Uric acid absorbs UV at 293 nm, although other compounds may also absorb at this wavelength. When urine samples are treated with uricase, uric acid is degraded into allantoin and other compounds that do not absorb UV at 293nm. Therefore, the reduction in OD reading after treatment with uricase is related with the concentration of uric acid in the sample. After treatment, OD of the standards should be zero if the conversion is complete.

Preparation of Standard
As in the case of xanthine. In this case also, prepare standard working concentration of 5, 10, 20, 30 and 40 mg/l.

Enzyme Preparation
Dilute the enzyme in the buffer to obtain a concentration of O. 12 U/ml (Uricase from Porcine liver: (Sigma Cat No. U-9375, 19 units/g solid). Keep the enzyme solution in the freeze to preserve the enzyme activity.

Procedure
a) Two sets of standards and a 'blank' (using distilled water) and samples in duplicate, are prepared.
b) Pipette 2.5 ml of urine or standard or water into 10 ml tubes.
c) Add 1 ml phosphate buffer (KH_2PO_4, 0.67M, pH 9.4 adjust the pH with KOH).
d) Mix well the contents of the tubes by Vortexing.
e) In one set, add 150 µl buffer and in the other add 150 µl of uricase solution

f) Mix again by vortexing and incubate in the water bath and 37°C for 90 min.
g) Remove from water bath, mix and transfer again the solutions to the cuvettes and read the OD at 293 nm. If the enzymatic conversion is complete, the OD of the standards with uricase added should be zero. If not, incubate in water bath for an additional 30 min. and read again.

Standard Curve and Calculations
a) Standard curve is curvilinear. When both X and Y are transformed to Ln functions, Ln (Y) is linearly correlated to Ln (X).
b) Use the OD reading of the set without addition of uricase for the construction of standard curve.
c) Calculate the net reduction in OD for the samples due to uricase treatment. OD = OD without enzyme - OD with enzyme.
d) Calculate the uric acid concentration from OD based on the established standard equation.

Calculations for Daily Excretion of Purine Derivatives
a) Calculate the excretion of allantoin, uric acid and xanthine plus hypoxanthine, unit of m mol/dl.
b) The total PD excretion (i.e. sum of all compounds) is used for the estimation of microbial protein supply.
c) In sheep the sum of all 4 compounds and in cattle the sum of allantoin and uric acid are taken into consideration. The proportion of the individual components expressed as % of the sum are approximately as follows.

In sheep = allantoin 60-80%; uric acid 30-10%, xanthin plus hypoxanthine 5 to 10%. As the total excretion increases, the proportion of allantoin increases. In cattle: Allantoin 80-85%, uric acid 15 to 20 % within the same animal, the proportions are very constant, but there seems to be variation between animals.

Calculation of Microbial N Supply

(A) Purine Absorption and PD Excretion

Different equations are used for sheep and cattle to describe the quantitative relationship between absorption of micrbial purines (X mmol/dl), and excretion of PD in urine(Y mmol/dl):

Sheep $Y = 0.84 X + (0.150 w^{0.75} e^{-0.25X})$ \hfill (1)
Cattle $Y = 0.85 X + (0.385 W^{0.75})$ \hfill (2)

Where $W^{0.75}$ represents the metabolic body weight (kg) of the animal. The slopes of 0.84 and 0.85 in; Equations (1) and (2) respectively, represent the recovery of absorbed purines as PD in urine. The component within parenthesis represents the net endogenous contribution of PD to total excretion after correction for the utilisation of microbial purines by the animal. In cattle, the endogenous contribution is taken as a constant at 0.385 mmol/kg $W^{0.75}$ per day. In sheep, this reduces to zero as exogenous purines are utilised and *de novo* synthesis of purines is phased out.

(B) Calculation of Daily Purine Absorption

Based on equations (1) and (2) above for sheep and cattle, respectively the amount of exogenous purines absorbed can then be estimated from the daily excretion of PD.

Sheep

The calculation of X from Y based on equation (1) can be performed by means of the Newton-Raphson iteration process, as shown below:

$$Xn_{+1} = \frac{Xn - f(Xn)}{F^{-1} - (Xn)} \quad (3)$$

Where,
$f(x) = 0.84 X + 0.150 W^{0.75} e^{-0.25x-y}$
And the derivatives of $f(x) = 0.84 - 0.038 W^{0.75} e^{-25x}$
Example = A sheep of 60 kg (W) excreted 5.0 mmol/d PD (Y). We give an initial value $X_1 = Y + 0.84 =$ to put in equation (3) to calculate X2, Now we obtain X2 = 4.838, Next we put X_2 back to equation (3) to calculate X_3 (X_3 = 4.790), and so on X4 and X5 can be calculated as 4.790 and 4.790, respectively. We will notice that, as the iteration process goes on, Xn approaches a constant value, which is the answer. In this example, the amount of microbial purines absorbed is therefore 4.79 mmol/dl.

Cattle

The calculation is straight forward
$X = (Y - 0.385 \times W^{0.75}) / 0.85 \quad (4)$
Example: A bull of 321 kg live weight, the daily excretion of purine derivatives was 153 mmol/dl. The amount of microbial purines absorbed can be calculated as: $(153 - 0.385 \times 321^{0.75}) / 0.85 = 145.7$ mmol/d.

(C) Calculation of Intestinal Flow of Microbial N

The following factors are used for the calculation of intestinal flow of microbial N (gN/d) from the microbial purines absorbed (X mmol/dl) (Equation 5).

(i) Digestibility of microbial purines is assumed to be 0.83.
(ii) This is taken as the mean digestibility value for microbial nucleic acids based on observations reported in the literature.
(iii) The N content of purines is 70 mgN/mmol.
(iv) The ratio of purine N: total N in mixed rumen microbes is taken as 11.6:100.

(v) Microbial N(gN/d) = $\dfrac{X \text{ (mmol/dl)} \times 70}{0.116 \times .83 \times 1000}$ = 0.727 x (5)

The results of the calculated microbial protein supply are expressed as "g" microbial N per day" and/or as " g microbial N per kg digestible organic matter intake (DOMI). The latter is effectively an expression of the efficiency of microbial protein supply. The efficiency can also be expressed as "g" microbial N per kg digestible organic matter apparently fermented in the rumen (DOMR). DOMR can be assumed to be 0.65 of the DOMI.

Purine derivatives (PD) concentration in plasma, their secretion in urine and milk ha long been considered as indicator for recovery of microbial protein available at duodenal level: which forms the major portion of metabolizable protein in ruminants (Mota *et al.*, 2008). The correlation of various nutrient utilization parameters with urinary PD excretion have been established already for eg. digestible dry matter (DDM) and organic matter (DOM) in ruminants (Chen et al., 1992 and Susmel *et. al.*, 1994); level of feed intake (Singh *et al.*, 2007) and levels of CP intake (Ramgaokar *et. al.*, 2008). So far, influence of energy levels on concentration of purine derivatives in different body fluids like milk, urine and plasma have not been studied in Indian dairy cattle. One of the recent studies claim that assay of allantoin and purine derivatives in milk samples can be used to assess the small variation in energy levels, and microbial protein supply of diets in dairy cattle (Deshpande *et. al.* 2011).

•••

Chapter 9

RUMEN FLUID VOLUME & ITS FLOW RATE

Principle

Polyethylene glycol (PEG) is a high molecular weight compound which is inert to rumen fermentation. The concentration in the rumen liquor declines with the passage of digesta from rumen to lower G.I. tract and is proportional to time. Protein free filtrate of rumen liquor gives turbidity in the presence of trichloro acetic acid and barium chloride which is a measure of PEG concentration at different post feeding hours.

Reagents

1. Polyethylene glycol (PEG) solution/(10%, w/v): 25g PEG (PEG 6000) is dissolved in distilled water to make volume 250 ml
2. Barium chloride (2.5%, w/v): Weigh 2.5g $BaCl_2$ and dissolve in distilled water to make volume 100 ml.
3. 0.3N $Ba(OH)_2$
4. 5% $ZnSO_4.7H_2O$: Dissolve 5g ZnSO4 $7H_2O$ in distilled water to make volume 100 ml
5. Trichloro acetic acid- Barium chloride solution: 5 g Barium chloride is dissolved in distilled water to make volume 100 ml. Then 25g trichloro acetic acid is added.
6. Standard PEG solution: Stock (1 mg/ml): weigh 100mg PEG and dissolve in distilled water to make final volume 100 ml.
7. Working standard (100 ug/ml.): Take 10 ml stock PEG solution and dilute with distilled water to make volume 100 ml.

Procedure

1. PEG solution (10%, w/v) is infused into the rumen at 4 different sites with the help of hard polythene tubes equipped with funnel on the top and multiple holes at the closed bottom, for dispersal of solution in all directions inside the rumen, The container and tube is given two washings for the transfer of PEG quantitatively.
2. The rumen contents are mixed thoroughly and strained rumen liquor (SRL) is collected from different sites at hourly interval (1,2,3,4,5,6,7,8h) upto 8h post feeding.
3. SRL is centrifuged at 5000 rpm for 15 min.
4. 2 ml supernatant SRL is taken in a test tube, into which 2 ml reagent 3, 2 ml reagent 4 and 4 ml reagent 2 are added.
5. The tube with the whole content (10ml) is shaken vigorously and allowed to stand for 5 min.
6. It is filtered through whatman No. 42 filter paper.
7. The filtrate, blank and the standard tubes are prepared as per the protocol given below.

Protocol

Reagent	Blank	Sample	Standard						
Distilled water (ml)	2.5	1.5	2.4	2.3	2.1	1.9	1.7	1.5
Standard PEG solution	-	-	0.1	0.2	0.4	0.6	0.8	1.0
Concentration of standard (μg)	-	-	10	20	40	60	80	100
Sample filtrate (ml)	-	1.0	-	-	-	-	-	-
Reagent (ml)	2.5	2.5	2.5	2.5	2.5	2.5	2.5	2.5

8. The tube with the contents are mixed thoroughly and the turbidity developed is measured at 540nm immediately after 20 min.
9. Plot a standard curve and the concentration of PEG at different hours post feeding (y) is plotted against time (x) to draw a regression line (y = a + bx). Concentration of PEG at 0h is obtained by extrapolating the graph to 0h.

Calculation

$$\text{Rumen fluid volume (I)} = \frac{\text{Amount PEG infused into the rumen (g)}}{\text{Concentration of PEG at 0h (g/ml)} \times 1000}$$

Rumen flow rate (t/h) = Rumen fluid volume (l) x exponential decline in PEG Concentration (slope b)

...

Chapter 10

CHROMATOGRAPHIC TECHNIQUES AND ITS APPLICATION IN ANIMAL NUTRITION RESEARCH

Nutrition plays a pivotal role for the animal research, be it health or production. Research in animal nutrition employs many basic techniques and chromatography is one of them. Chromatographic processes can be defined as separation techniques involving mass transfer between stationary and mobile phases. Various types of chromatography have one application or the other in analysis of food/feed components (Day and Williamson, 2001), quantitation of nutrients as well as the characterization of the effect of nutrients in biological samples like serum/plasma or tissues (Merken and Beecher, 2000).

A. Principle

Basically all chromatographic systems consist of the **stationary phase** that may be solid, gel, liquid or a solid/liquid mixture that is immobilized and the mobile phase, which may be gas or liquid and it flows over or through the stationary phase. This partition is achieved in one of the following ways:

Adsorption chromatography : It is one of the oldest types of chromatography. It utilizes a mobile liquid or a gaseous phase that is adsorbed onto the surface of a stationary solid phase. The equilibrium between the mobile and the stationary phase accounts the separation of different solutes e.g. adsorption chromatography, hydrophobic interaction chromatography.

Partition chromatography : It is based on a thin film formed on the surface of a solid support by a liquid stationary phase. Solutes equilibrate between the mobile and the stationary liquid (e.g. partition chromatography, reverse phase chromatography, gas-liquid chromatography, etc.).

Ion exchange chromatography: In this type, the use of a resin as the stationary solid phase, to covalently attach anions or cations onto it. Solute ions of the opposite charge in the mobile liquid phase are attracted to the resin by electrostatic forces (e.g. ion-exchange chromatography, chromatofocussing).

Molecular exclusion chromatography : This gel permeation chromatography lacks an attractive interaction between the stationary phase and the solute. The liquid or the gaseous phase passes through a porous gel which separates the molecules according to size. The pores are normally small and exclude the larger solute molecules, but allows smaller molecules to enter the gel, causing them the flow through a larger volume. This causes the larger molecules to pass through the column at a faster rate than the smaller ones (e.g. gel aeration chromatography).

Affinity chromatography : This is the most selective type of chromatography employed. It utilizes the specific interaction between one kind of solute molecules and a second molecule that is immobilized on a stationary phase. For example, the immobilized ligand may be an antibody to some protein. When solute containing a mixture of proteins are passed by this ligand, only the specific protein is reacted to this antibody, binding it to the stationary phase. This protein is later extracted by changing the ionic strength or pH.

B. Modes of chromatography
Chromatographic separations can be achieved in three ways.

Paper chromatography : Here stationary liquid phase is supported by the cellulose fibres of a paper sheet. Mobile phase passes along the paper sheet either by gravity (descending paper chromatography) or by capillary action (ascending paper chromatography). This is one of the oldest forms of chromatography. Although, it is not much aplicable today, still it used to demonstrate the principle of chromatography. Eg. Separation of amino acids in a mixture.

Thin layer chromatography: In TLC, the stationary phase attached to a suitable matrix is coated thinly onto a glass, plastic or metal foil surface.

The mobile liquid phase passes across the thin layer plate held either horizontally or vertically, by capillary action. This mode of chromatography has the advantage that many samples can be studied simultaneously. Eg. separation of neutral lipids, phospholipids or sugars in a mixture.

Column chromatography: The process of chromatographic separation takes place within a column. This column made of glass or metal is either a packed bed or open tubular column. A packed bed column contains particles which make up the stationary phase. Open tubular columns are lined with a thin film stationary phase. The centre of the column is hollow. The mobile phase is typically a solvent moving through the column which carries the mixture to be separated. This mobile phase can be a liquid (Liquid chromatography) or a gas (gas chromatography).

The stationary phase is usually a viscous liquid coated on the surface of solid particles which are packed into the column although, solid particles can also be taken as a stationary phase. In any case, partitioning of solutes between the stationary and mobile phases leads to the desired separation.

C. Basic operation of column chromatography

The process involves 4 steps.

Feed injection : The feed is injected into the mobile phase which flows through the system by the action of a pump (older techniques used capillary action or gravity to move the mobile phase).

Separation in the column : As the sample flows through the column, its different components will adsorb to the stationary phase to varying degrees. Those with strong attraction to the support move more slowly than those with weak atrractions. This is how components are separated.

Elution from the column : After the sample is displaced from the stationary phase, the different components will elute from the column at different times. The components with the least affinity for the stationary phase (the most weakly adsorbed) will elute first, while those with the greatest affinity for the stationary phase (the most strongly adsorbed) will elute last.

Detection: The different components are detected as they emerge from the column-A detector analyzes the emerging stream by measuring a property which is related to concentration and characteristics of chemical composition. For example, the refractive index or ultra-violet absorbance is measured.

The output from the detector is the **chromatogram** representing separate peak for different component separated from a sample mixture. The following infprmation can be drawn from the chromatogram.

i) The level of complexity of the sample is indicated by the number of peaks which appear. A purified component will reveal one sharp peak on chromatogram.
ii) Qualitative information about the sample composition is obtained by comparing peak positions with those of standards.
iii) Quantitative assessment of the relative concentrations of components is obtained from peak area comparisons.
iv) Characterization of the components by comparing with a set of standards.
v) Column performance is indicated by comparison with standards.

D. Gas chromatography

Gas chromatography makes use of a pressurized gas cylinder and a carrier gas, such as helium, to carry the solute through the column. The most common detector used in this type of chromatography are thermal conductivity and flame ionization detectors. There are three types of gas chromatography. .

Gas adsorption chromatography : It involves a packed bed comprised of an adsorbent used as a stationary phase. Common adsorbents are zeolite, silica gel and activated alumina. This method is commonly used to separate a mixture of gases

Gas-liquid chromatography : It is more common type of analytical chromatography. In this type of column, an inert porous solid is coated with a viscous liquid which acts as a stationary phase. Diatomous earth is the most common solid used. Solutes in the feed stream dissolve into the liquid phase and eventually vaporize. The separation is thus based on relative volatilities e.g. analysis of fatty acid composition in a mixture.

Capillary gas chromatography : It is the most common analytical method. Glass or fused silica comprise the capillary walls which are coated with an absorbent or other solvent. Because of the small amount of the stationary phase, the column can contain only a limited capacity. This method also yields a rapid separation of mixtures.

E. Liquid chromatography

It was first discovered in 1903 by M.S. Tswelt, who used a chalk column to separate the pigments of green leaves. Only in 1960s, the more emphasis was placed on the development of liquid chromatography. There are a variety of types of liquid chromatography. Modern liquid chromatography includes the following types.

Reverse phase chromatography : It is a powerful analytical tool and involves a hydrophobic, low polarity stationary phase which is chemically bonded to an inert solid such as silica. The separation is essentially an extraction operation and is useful for separating non-volatile compounds.

Size exclusion chromatography : It does not involve adsorption and is extremly fast. The packing is a porous gel of dextran (sephadex, sephacryl), agarose (sepharose, Biogel A) or polyacrylamide (Biogel P). The gel is capable of separating molecules on the basis of size. The larger molecules elute first since they cannot penetrate the pores. This method is common in protein separation and purification.

High performance liquid chromatography (HPLC) : It is most widely used analytical technique. HPLC utilizes a liquid mobile phase to separate the components of a mixture. These components (or analytes) are first dissolved in a solvent, then forced to flow through a chromatographic column under a high pressure. In the column, the mixture is resolved into its components. The amount of resolution is important and it is dependent upon the extent of interaction between the solute components and the stationary phase (immobile packing material in the column). The interaction of the solute with two phases can be manipulated through different choices of both solvents and stationary phases. As a result, HPLC acquires a high degree of versatility not found in other chromatographic systems and it has the ability to easily separate a wide variety of chemical mixtures. HPLC as compared with classical chromatography technique is characterized by :

(i) Small diameter (2.5 mm), reusable stainless steel columns.
(ii) Column packings with very small (3, 5 and 10 mm) particles and the continual development of new substances to be used as stationary phases.
(iii) Relatively high inlet pressures and controlled flow of mobile phases.
(iv) Precise sample introduction without the need for large samples.
(v) Special continuous flow detectors capable of handling small flow rates and detecting very small amounts.
(vi) Automated standardized instruments.
(vii) Rapid analysis and

(viii) High resolution.

The high performance is the result of many factors, very small particles of narrow distribution range and uniform pore size and distribution, high pressure column packing techniques, accurate low volume sample injectors, sensitive low volume detectors and good pumping systems. Pressure is needed to permit a given flow rate of mobile phase only.

Type of HPLC

On the basis of the nature of stationary and the mobile phase, HPLC can be classified into adsorption, partition, ion exchange and size exclusion chromatography where the principle is mentioned before and the suitable stationary phase and the support is used.

Concerning the adsorption chromatography, two modes can be defined depending on the relative polarity of the two phases.

Normal phase chromatography : The stationary bed is strongly polar in nature (e.g. silica gel) and the mobile phase is non polar (such as n-hexane or tetrahydrofuran). Polar samples are thus retained on the polar surface of the column packing longer than the less polar materials.

Reverse phase chromatography: Stationary bed is nonpolar (hydrophobic) in nature, while the mobile phase is a polar liquid, such as mixture of water and methanol or acetonitrile. More nonpolar the material is, the longer it will be retained.

Eluent polarity plays the highest role in separation. In all types of HPLC, there are two elution types:

Isocratic elution : Constant eluent composition is pumped through the column during whole analysis.

Gradient elution : Eluent composition (and strength) is steadily changed during the run.

F. Selection of a chromatographic system

The types of the system most likely to be applicable depends on the physical characteristics of the compound under separation as most of the chromatographic techniques are based upon the differences in the physical properties of compounds in a mixture. Some of the guidelines are as follows.
1. Volatile compounds are best separated by GLC. Recent developments in capillary gas chromatography make it a sensitive system for volatile compounds. Mass spectrometry coupled with GC provides the most

useful tool for identification of the separated compounds.
2. Non-volatile compounds that are soluble in organic solvents can be easily separated either by adsorption or by normal phase chromatography. The compounds having different functional groups can be separated by adsorption chromatography on silica with nonpolar solvents. Low polarity compounds in a homologous series are separated by normal phase chromatography.
3. Non-ionic or weakly ionic water soluble compounds are preferably separated by reverse-phase chromatography.
4. Strongly ionic water soluble compounds are best separated by ion exchange chromatography using cationic or anionic resin depending upon the charge of the protein.
5. Compounds having different size are isolated using gel filteration chromatography.
6. HPLC is a powerful, fast and precise technique for qualitative and quantitative separation and also characterization of the compounds. However, the use of HPLC depends on many factors including availability of the apparatus, cost and the scale of separation. HPLC-MS is most useful for identification of the compounds.
7. If the compound to be separated has ligand binding property, affinity chromatography is a method of choice

Chapter 11

FRACTIONATION OF VOLATILE FATTY ACIDS WITH GAS LIQUID CHROMATOGRAPHY

Chromatography is one of the most effective technique for accurate, fast and convenient separation and identification of the components of a mixture. The method was developed by Russian botanist Mikhail Tswett (1906), described by Karl Runge (1855). Martin and Synage (1944) received Noble Prize for developing methodology of partition Chromatography.

Partition chromatography
Partition chromatogaphy is a system comprising of two physically distinguished components - a mobile component or phase and a stationary component or phase. A mixture of substances which are to be separated is placed on the system and separation takes place on the basis of difference in distribution of molecular species in two phases. Relative movement is a result of driving force and retarding effects.

Stationary phase is the sorbent, which may be liquid or paper or gel. If it is liquid then it is held stationary by adsorbing on a solid support or matrix. The mobile phase may be solvent or developer or a gas. Since the two phases are immiscible, the partitioning is defined as the distribution of solute in two immisicible phases which are in contact with one another. When a column is filled with the sorbent and solvent the two phases form a large number of theoretical plates. Each plate contains both the phases. Solutes in solution (mixture of substances to be separated) is layered on the top of the column and when it enters to the column it distributes in the two phases. The ratio of the concentration of a solute in two phases is called its partition coefficient. The resolution of solutes improves as the length of stationary phase increases.

Gas liquid chromatography (GLC)

The chromatography system is termed as gas liquid chromatography because here stationary phase is a liquid and mobile phase is a gas. The whole unit of GLC comprises of :

Injector : For loading of sample on the column.
Column : Tubing (glass or stainless steel) packed with stationary phase.
Detector : For measuring the quantity of separated components. There are two types of detectors, Flame Ionization Detector (F.I.D.) and Thermal Conductivity Detector (T.C.D.).
Oven and
Heaters : For temperature control of column, detector and injector.
Carrier gas : To provide a suitable gas flow through the column which can take with them the components of the mixture. The commonly used carrier gases are nitrogen, hydrogen, argon and helium.

A sample is injected into the column along with carrier gas near the head of packed chromatographic column. Separation of various components of the sample occurs as a result of multiple forces by which the column material tend to retain these components. In the gas phase the components move towards the outlet, but they are selectively retarded by the stationary phase. Consequently, all components pass through the column at varying speeds and emerge in the inverse order of their retention by the column material. Upon emerging from the column, the gaseous phase immediately enters a detector attached to the column. Here the individual components register a series of signals which appear as peaks on the chromatogram. The chromatographic peaks are used for qualitative and quantitative detection of the components.

Qualitative analysis

Qualitative analysis (identification of the components) of the components in a mixture can be done on the basis of fact, that each component has a characteristic retention time in the column when passing through the column in a particular operating conditions. By comparing the chromatogram of the sample with the chromatogram of the mixture of the known components assumed to be present in the sample, the components of the sample can be identified by comparing the retention time.

Quantitative analysis

A typical chromatogram consists of a baseline and the peaks. The distance between peaks is influenced by the rate of flow of gas, the column conditions and column temperature. However, peak area is related to the concentration of component. On the basis of the fact, a calibration curve is necessary which can be prepared by using a mixture of known concentrations of known components as a standard. A comparison between a calibration curve with that of sample will tell about the concentration of a component.

Conditions for fractionation of volatile fatty acids on GLC

A mixture of volatile fatty acids can be fractionated on GLC, by using following conditions:
1. The detector in Flame Ionization Detector (F.I.D.)
2. Column is packed with cromosorb 101 and the size of the column is 1.8 mm diameter and 4 feet length.
3. Flow rate
   - Nitrogen   30ml/min (carrier gas)
   - Hydrogen   30ml/min
   - Air   320ml/min
4. Temperature
   - Injector oven 270°C
   - Column oven   172°C
   - Detector oven 270°C
5. Sample size   1µl

Conditioning of column

The conditioning of column should be done at every 8 to 10 days interval or if base line is not adjusting by running the GLC for 6 to 8h without sample, keeping the following conditions. The flow of gases are to be kept same as above.
- Oven   240°C
- Injector   260°C
- Detector   260°C

Preparation of sample

Draw rumen liquor from a cannulated animal and filter it through 4 layers of muslin cloth. Take 5ml of strained rumen liquor, add to it 1 ml metaphosphoric acid (25%). Metaphosphoric acid precipitates the proteins which contaminate the column. Stand the sample for 30 minutes and then centrifuge it at 4000 rpm for 20 minutes. Collect the clear supernatant and use for analysis.

Preparation of standard

Stock solutions of individual acids

Acetic acid: Take 250 mg acetic acid in a volumetric flask and make it to 10ml with distilled water. The concentration of the solution is 25 mg/ml

Propionic acid: Take 250 mg propionic acid in a volumetric flask and make it to 10ml with distilled water. The concentration of the solution is 25 mg/ml.

Iso-butyric acid: Take 250 mg iso-butyric acid in a volumetric flask and make it to 10 ml with distilled water. The concentration of the solution is. 25 mg/ml.

Butyric acid: Take 250 mg butyric acid in a volumetric flask and make it to 10ml with distilled water. The concentration of the solution is 25 mg/ml.

Iso-valeric acid: Take 250 mg iso-valeric acid in a volumetric flask and make it to 10 ml with distilled water. The concentration of the solution is 25 mg/ml.

Valerie acid: Take 250 mg valeric acid in a volumetric flask and make it to 10 ml with distilled water. The concentration of the solution is 25 mg/ml.

Working Standard mixture of acids (10 ml.)

Acid	ml acid / 10ml. mix	Final Concentration	
		(mg/ml.)	(mm/CO and)
Acetic acid	1.68	4.2	7.00
Propionic acid	0.48	1.2	1.62
Inobutynic acid	0.12	0.3	0.34
Butynic acid	0.24	0.6	0.68
Irovalenic acid	0.12	0.3	0.29
Valenic acid	0.12	0.3	0.29
Distilled water	Make the volume to 10 ml		

Precautions
1. A sample size should not be bigger than 1µl for liquids and 1 cc for gases to get good resolution.
2. Oven temperature should be usually 50°C above the normal boiling point of the sample.
3. Injector temperature should be 25°C to 50°C above that of the column

oven temperature for the best results
4. When dual Column system is used, the flow rate should be same in both the columns to get best results.
5. After using the columns, it should be washed by injecting acetone into the column at least twice to remove any left over of the samples.
6. Instrument should be switched off sequentially in the reverse order as it was started.
7. Supply of carrier gas to the instrument should be stopped only when the column and detector temperature has fallen to near ambient temperature. Column should not be allowed to remain in a heated oven without a flow of carrier gas, it will spoil the column.
8. There should not be any leakage in the gas supply system.
9. Gases of high purity should be used.
10. Instrument should be kept in dirt free clean place.

Estimation of methane by GLC

Conditions for methane estimation

1. The detector is Flame Ionization Detector (EI.D.).
2. Column is Porapak-Q
3. Flow rate
   Nitrogen   30 ml/min (carrier gas)
   Hydrogen   30 ml/min
   Air   300 ml/min
4. Temperature
   Injector oven   40°C
   Column oven   50°C
   Detector oven   50°C
5. Sample size   25 µl

Standard
The standard gas for methane estimation consists of 50% methane and 50% carbon. Of this mixture 25 µl is injected in the column i.e. 12.5 µl of methane.

Sample
The gas produced in the fermentation vessel can be directly used for methane estimation. With the help of gas tight syringe, inject 100 µl gas. Care should be taken that no water traces should enter the column.

Area of internal standard

Procedure
1. Switch on Gas Chromatograph sequentially in the following manner
   a. Check every switch in off position
   b. Adjust the flow rate of the three gasses one by one with the help of soap bubble meter.
   c. Light the flame
   d. Switch on the temperature controller module and feed the required temperatures.
   e. Switch on F. I. D. module.
   f. Allow the system to stabilize.
2. Make repeat 1.0µl injections of the composite working standard until a stable response is obtained. Under these conditions, the analysis of rumen liquor takes about 10min from acetic to valeric acid.
3. Now inject 1µl of sample and have chromatogram of the sample.

Calculations
Calculate mg/ml of each acid in the strained rumen liquor from the Expression:

Conc. of unknown = RF_1 x standard conc. x df x RF_2

Where,

$$RF_1 = \frac{\text{Area of sample component peak}}{\text{Area of internal standard}}$$

$$RF_2 = \frac{\text{Area of known peak}}{\text{Area of internal statement}}$$

df = Dilution factor

•••

Chapter 12

HIGH PERFORMANCE LIQUID CHROMATOGRAPHIC ANALYSIS OF KARANJIN IN KARANJ (HONGE) SEED CAKE

Various products of karanj (Pongamia glabra) are utilized for industrial, health and animal agricultural application in the Indian subcontinent. Despite a rich source of protein (CP 28 —34 %), karanj (honge) cake is found to be slightly bitter in taste and toxic owing to the presence of furanoflavonoid (Karanjin), restricting its safe inclusion in the livestock diets. Though a non polar solvent, soxhlet extraction of karanj seed cake with petroleum ether/ acetone drastically reduces karanjin content. The residual cake left after solvent extraction is proved to be safe as animal feed supplement.

Estimation of karanjin
The samples can be analysed for the toxin, karanjin as per the method of Prabhu *et al.* (2002).

Extraction of Karanjin from Raw and Processed Cake
Exactly 25 gm of ground and thoroughly mixed sample is weighed and transferred into the thimble and extracted for 12h using 200ml of freshly distilled methanol as solvent. Methanol extract is then cooled and filtered into preweighted round bottom flask using Whatman No.1 filter paper. The excess methanol is distilled off under vacuum. The flask containing the extract is weighed again to obtain the weight of extract by subtracting the

empty flask's weight. Sufficient amount of moisture free extract is transferred into vials for further analysis.

Apparatus
The liquid chromatograph fitted with P- 2000 pumping system and UV-150 series detector and silica gel prepacked analytical column (RP-18, 7 µm)

Solvents and Elution
Solvents are filtered using a glass Millipore system with a 0.45 µm filter and degassed at room temperature under vacuum with magnetic stirring. Working solutions containing 10mg of sample per 1 ml of methanol are filtered through a swinny stainless unit with a 0.45 µm filter. The elution solvent system consisted of methanol and water (80:20) run at a flow rate of 1 ml/min and at an average pressure of 2000 p.s.i. Samples are dissolved and injected on to the column using a micro-injector (20µl).

Detction : The UV detector is set at 250 nm.

Method to calculate the content of karanjin
Area points are taken into consideration to calculate the karanjin levels and following formulae are used to express the karanjin content in percentages.

a) $x \text{ ppm} = \dfrac{\text{Area point of test}}{\text{Area point of standard}}$

b) Karanjin content in methanol extract $= \dfrac{x}{10,000} \times 100\% = \dfrac{x}{100} \%$

c) Karanjin content in treatment $= x \times \dfrac{x}{100} = \dfrac{y}{100} = \dfrac{xx}{10,000}$

x = Karanjin in ppm
y = % methanol extract

Chapter 13

ESTIMATION OF AZADIRACHTIN IN NEEM SEED CAKE BY HPLC

Neem seed cake (NSC) despite of being rich in protein is not used as animal feed due to the presence of large number of toxic/bitter compounds in it. Studies have shown that NSC can be safely included the ration of animals after water washing / alkali/ urea treatment. These treatment methods appear to remove / reduce or largely inactivate the toxic principles present in NSC. In order to assess the quality/safety of the treated product, quantification of the residual toxic compounds is essential. One such compound is azadirachtin. It has been reported to be biologically most active.

One of the best techniques for the estimation of azadirachtin is by using high performance liquid chromatography (HPLC).

Equipment
i) HPLC with isocratic or quaternary pump fitted with injection valve, degasser, C_{18} ODS column, PDA detector, monitor, integrator etc.
ii) Rotary vacuum evaporator
iii) Vacuum pump

Glassware: separating funnels, beakers, conical flask, filtration assembly, sintered funnels and chromatographic columns.
Chemicals: solvents—petroleum ether, methanol, dichloromethane, diethyl ether, acetone (LR, AR and HPLC grade).
Silica gel and pure azadirachtin (Sigma)
Other material : membrane filters, syringe, syringe filters.

Preparation of sample :

1. Removal fat/oil

Grind 1 kg of neem seed cake in a mixer-cum-grinder to a fine powder. Add one liter of petroleum ether / hexane and agitate for 10 min. in the mixer-cum-grinder. Transfer the material to a 5 liter conical flask and allow to settle for 12 hours. Then agitate the mixture again in the mixer for 5 min. Filter the resulting suspension through a large Buchner funnel under vacuum. After filtration, transfer the extracted cake to the blender and agitate again in 1 liter of petroleum ether for five min. and filter through Buchner funnel. Repeater this process 3-4 times to remove the oily portion as much as possible. This fraction contains very little of AZADIRACHTIN. It can be used for estimation of salannin after vaccum drying

2. Extraction of azadirachtin

Petroleum ether extract of NSC is treated with 95% ethyl alcohol then it is transferred to 5 liter conical flask and allowed to stand for 12 hours. Filter the solvent through Buchner funnel under pressure. Remove the solvent by rotary vacuum evaporator. A dark viscous extract (approx. 71g) will be obtained.

Then partition the ethanolic extract 2 times between petroleum ether and aqueous methanol (66%) to remove the remaining oil and other non — polar materials. Collect this non-polar — fraction (F_1). Again partition the aqueous methanol fraction against dichloromethane to remove water-soluble protein and sugars. Collect dichloromethane (F_2) and aqueous methanol fractions (F_3) separately. Azadirachtin is largely present in dichloromethane (F_2) fraction.

3. Column chromatography

Reduce the volume of fraction F_2 to about 25 ml by rotary vacuum evaporator. Add weighed quantity of silica gel (column chromatography grade, mesh 60-240) for coating with the extract by tumbling in the rotary evaporator. Weigh the coated material and load it at the top of silica gel column (10g). Elute successively with about 80-100 ml of light petroleum ether (60-80° C) (F_4), petroleum ether and diethyl ether (80:20 by volume) (F_5); diethyl ether (100%) (F_6), diethyl ether + acetone (80:20)(F_7) and finally with methanol (100%) (F_8). Reduce the volume of fractions 4-8 by rotary vacuum evaporation and collect the concentrated material for the estimation of azadirachtin by HPLC.

HPLC Determination of azadirachtin

Standarzation & calibration

Stock solution : Dissolve known quantity (20 µg) of pure azadirachtin (Sigma grade) in 2 ml of HPLC grade methanol.

Working standard solution: take 5, 10, 20 and 500µl of the stock solution and make up the volume to 1000 with HPLC grade methanol (60%).

Calibration of HPLC instrument : Inject 20µl of each of the above working standard azadirachtin solution to test the linearity and detection limit of the instrument at 217 nm. Note the retention time.

Analysis of the sample : Dissolve different fractions i.e. F_4 to F_8 in methanol. Inject 20µl of the unknown sample. Use 60:40 methanol: water as mobile phase at a stable flow rate of 0.75 ml/min. Take the calibration at 217 nm. Record the peaks and compare it with the standard.

Calculation : The concentration of azadirachtin can be calculated from the peak area as follows :

$$\text{Azadirachtin content (\%)} = \frac{A_1 \times M_2 \times P}{A_2 \times M_1} \times 100$$

Where,
A_1 = peak area of unknown sample solution
A_2 = peak are of azadirachtin in reference standard solution
M_1 = mass in gram of test sample
M_2 = mass in gram of the reference standard azadirachtin
P = purity of reference standard azadirachtin (%)

Result : Azadirachtin content in different fractions are expressed in percentage unit.

Chapter 14

ESTIMATION OF RICIN IN CASTOR BEAN MEAL BY SDS-PAGE

In spite of its high protein (CP, 34-36%) content, castor bean meal as such is not used as livestock feed due to the presence of toxic factors viz., ricin, ricinine and allergen. Of the three, ricin is the most detrimental to animals. In order to detoxify the castor cake, a number of physical and chemical methods are employed. The efficacy of the treatments is assessed, based on the qualitative and quantitative changes in ricin content. Of all the detoxification methods, autoclaving (15 p.s.i., 60 min) and lime (4% w/w) treatments completely destroy the toxin. (Anandan *et. al.*, 2005).

Estimation of Ricin

The raw and detoxified samples can be analysed for the toxin, ricin as per the method of Kabat *et al.* (1947) with modifications as suggested by Waller and Negi (1958).

Extraction of Ricin

The solvent extracted castor cake sample of 500 g is extracted with 2.5 l of water acidified with HCl to a pH of 3.8 by shaking the contents in a conical flask for 6 h. The contents are allowed to settle and are then filtered trough Whatman filter paper No.1 . The residue is treated with 1.5 l of distilled water, shaken for 3 h and filtered through the same paper. A second treatment with water is given to the residue and filtered again through the same filterpaper.

This filtrate contains all the ricin and portions of ricinine that are soluble in cold, dilute HCI. It is evaporated to a small volume by vacuum distillation below 40 °C. The filtrate is saturated with sodium chloride and centrifuged at 4000 rpm for 20 min. to separate the precipitate containing only ricin.

Purification of ricin

The precipitate is dissolved in deionised and distilled water. It is reprecipitated at pH 8 by saturation with ammonium sulphate. After reprecipitation twice more with the same salt, they are dissolved in deionisel water and dialyzed at 4°C for a period of 72 h against tris buffer adjusted to pH 6.8 using dialysis membrane- 110(HIMEDIA). The buffer is changed once in 2h for the first 12 h and subsequently once in 6 h for the remaining period.

After 72 h, the dialysate is centrifuged at 4000 rpm for 10 min to separate the insoluble matter from the clear solution containing ricin. The solution is concentrated under vacuum and the amount of solution is measured. The ricin is estimated as the quantity of protein present in the dialysate as per the method of Lowry *et al.* (1951). The extract of the castor cake obtained after dialysis are subjected to SDS-PAGE (sodium dodecyl sulphate polyacrylamide gel electrophoresis) as per the method (Laemmli, 1970) for qualitative determination of ricin.

Sodium Dodecyl Sulphate Polyacrylamide Gel Electrophoresis (SDS-PAGE) Analysis of Extracted Ricin

The ricin obtained after dialysis is subjected to denaturing — PAGE analysis using sodium dodecyl sulphate as a denaturing agent. An extract from untreated castor cake (control) equivalent to 50 µg protein and protein (ricin extracted and purified) from treated material on an equivalent basis to the amount of untreated cake that yielded 50 µg protein are mixed with sample buffer containing 20ml mercapto-ethanol and 200ml glycerol per liter of 0.5 M tris HCl (pH 6.8) to make 40 µl volume and loaded in each well. Proteins are separated in 12.5 % acrylamide gel (10 cm x 10cm x 0.1cm) prepared as per the method of Laemmli (1970) on which 5% stacking gel (4cm x 10 cm x 0.1cm) is layered. Electrophoresis condition is set at 40 V till the dye front reached the separating gel and then fixed at 60 V till the sample reached the end. After complete run, protein is fixed for 1 h in a solution containing methanol (500ml) and acetic acid (100ml) and then stained overnight using a solution containing coomassie brilliant blue-R dye (2.5 g), methanol (400ml) and acetic acid (100ml). The protein bands in the gel are visualized by destaining using a solution containing methanol (250ml) and acetic acid (70ml). Molecular weights of the stained bands of extracted ricin in control and treated cake are determined using known molecular weight marker (Sigma, USA.)

•••

Chapter 15

UV VISIBLE SPECTROPHOTOMETRIC METHOD OF ESTIMATION OF GOSSYPOL

Cotton *(Gossypium)* seed meal (CSM), the by-product of cotton seed oil industry, is widely used as an animal feed. However, its utilization as an animal feed is limited due to the presence of gossypol, a polyphenolie binaphthyl aldyde, which is toxic to non-ruminants such as poultry and swine and young ruminants such as calves and lambs. The gossypol (free gossypol, FG) present primarily in the pigment glands of cotton seed, is mostly converted to bound gossypol due to condensation of aldehyde group with free amino groups of proteins to form a schiff base. Formation of schiff base though results in the detoxification of gossypol to some extent, it also lowers the nutritive value by reducing the availability of lysine, the limiting amino acid of cotton seed. Thus, bound gossypol, consequently total gossypol (TG) (free plus bound) content is an important factor of cotton seed meal.

Principle

Total gossypol

The method for total gossypol estimation involves oxalic acid hydrolysis of the bound gossypol in a methyl ethyl ketone-water azeotrope, partitioning the liberated gossypol into chloroform and quantification by second derivative UV spectrophotometry at 300 nm which permits direct quantification of all compounds containing nepthalene nuclei, chromogenic reaction is not required (SD, 4.0%; overall recovery, 89.5%).

Free gossypol

The method of free gossypol estimation involves extraction of free gossypol by aqueous acetone hydrolysis of the soluble forms of gossypol with hydrochloric acid, partitioning of the pure compound into chloroform and analysis by derivative UV spectrophotometry at 300 nm, the reactions requiring no chromogenic reagent (SD, 4.0%; overall accuracy, 91.2%).

Reagents
(a) Aquous acetone :
    Mix 700 ml acetone with 300 ml glass distilled water.
(b) Methyl ethyl ketone-water-azeotrope:
    Mix 1106 ml reagent grade methyl ethyl ketone with 110 ml water and distilled, rejecting the first 100ml of distillate. Azeotrope distills at 73.5°C. Store in brown bottle.
(c) Oxalic acid solution 0.1 M :
    Dissolve 12.6g oxalic acid dihydrate in 1000 ml methyl ethyl ketone-water azeotrope and store in brown bottle.
(d) Solvent mixture:
    Mix 715 ml ethanol, 285 ml distilled water, 200 ml peroxide free diethyl ether and 2 ml reagent grade glacial acetic acid. Store in brown bottle.
(e) Other chemicals:
    Chloroform, sodium sulphate and hydrochloric acid.
(f) Gossypol stock solution :
    Weigh accurately 12 mg of standard gossypol-acetic acid (89.62% gossypol by weight; Sigma chemicals) and dissolve in 50 ml solvent mixture. Aliquots of stock solution are further diluted to give working solutions in the range of 0.7-4 µg/ml. Stock and working solutions are prapared daily and protected from light throughout the analysis.

Apparatus required
1. Double beam UV-Visible spectrophotometer with 10 mm quartz absorption cells.
2. Water bath
3. Rotary vacuum evaporator
4. Laboratory mill equipped with 1 mm screen.
5. Wrist action mechanical shaker.

Standard curve for total and free gossypol
Measure optical density (O.D.) of working solutions at 300 nm. Plot calibration curve taking concentration of gossypol (µg/ml) on x-axis against corresponding O.D. on Y-axis.
[Regression of gossypol (mg/ml) concentration (y) on O.D. (x) revealed a linear response within the observed range with a correlation co-efficient (r) of 0.999 giving a model equation.
Y=0.006315 + 39.7326X; where X = O.D. and Y = gossypol concentration (µg/ml)

Sample preparation
Grind approximately 50g cotton seed meal in laboratory mill through 1 mm screen. Care should be taken to avoid overheating and oil expression while grinding, especially when seeds are ground.

Procedure

(A) Estimation of total gossypol:
Accurately weigh 1g of ground CSM into 100 ml volumetric flask and add 25 ml oxalic acid solution. Place flask in 75°C water bath, allow to equilibrate, then stopper flask and heat for 6 hours. Remove flask from water bath, cool to room temperature and add 25 ml aqueous acetone followed by 5 ml barium acetate solution. Mix minimum contents of flask and dilute to volume with aqueous acetone. Let stand 10 min. for complete precipitation of formed barium oxalate and filter through Whatman No. 41 filter paper into glass-stopper flask, discarding first 10 ml of filtrate. Pipet 25 ml aliquot of filtered extract into 250 ml separatory tunnel and add 50 ml chloroform followed by 100 ml distilled water acidified with 1 ml hydrochloric acid. Shake funnel 3 min to accomplish partitioning, let stand 5 min. and filter lower organic layer through anhydrous sodium sulphate on Whatman No. 40 filter paper into 100 ml glass stoppered round bottom flask. Rinse sodium sulphate by filtering through filter paper with 10 ml chloroform and evaporate filtrate to dryness in vacuum evaporator at 40°C. Dissolve dried residue with 25 ml solvent mixture in stopper flask.

Pipet appropriate sample solution into 10 ml volumetric flask and dilute to volume with solvent mixture. Size of aliquot depends on total gossypol content of sample : for sample with expected total gossypol content <3000 ppm, use> 1.0 ml aliquot; 3000-5000 ppm, 1 ml aliquot; 5000-7000 ppm, 0.7 ml aliquot; 7000-9000 ppm, 0.6 ml aliquot; 9000-11000 ppm 0.5 ml aliquot and 11000-13000 ppm. 0.4 ml aliquot. For maximum precision, resulting final solution should contain about 2.5 µg gossypol/ml. Read O.D. of final solution against solvent mixture at 300 nm.

Calculations

Calculate total gossypol content of CSM as follows:
Total gossypol, ppm = (2000 x C) / (V x W)
Where,
C = gossypol concentration (mg/ml) of final solution from standard curve,
V = volume of aliquot taken (ml), and
W = weight of sample (g)

(B) Estimation of free gossypol:

Estimation of free gossypol involves extraction, hydrolysis and clean up procedures.

Extraction : Transfer an accurately weighed sample of ground (1mm screen) cotton seed meal (3g) to a 250ml glass stoppered Erlenmeyer flask after covering the bottom of flask with glass beads (4mm diameter). Add 100 ml of 70% aqueous acetone and shake the flask for 1 hour on a wrist action mechanical shaker. Filter the contents of flask through Whatman No. 40 filter paper into another flask, after discarding first 5 ml of filtrate.

Hydrolysis and clean up

Pipet 2 ml of aliquot of filtrate into a 50 ml volumetric flask and add 1 drop (0.5ml) of hydrochloric acid. Heat the flask contents on a water bath at 65°C for 1 hour and cool it to room temperature. Transfer the contents to a 250 ml separatory funnel with two rinses, 3 ml each, of 70% aqueous acetone. Add 100 ml of acidified (1ml hydrochloric acid) distilled water into the funnel. Extract the formed suspension with 50 ml of chloroform and filter lower organic layer through anhydrous sodium sulphate on Whatman No. 40 filter paper into a 100 ml glass stoppered round bottom flask. Rinse sodium sulphate and filter paper with an additional 5 ml of chloroform. Evaporate the filtrate to dryness in a vacuum oven at 35°C. Dissolve the dried residue with 25 ml solvent mixture and store in the flask until analysed. Values of gossypol are unchanged on standing upto 6 hours.

Read O.D. of sample solution against solvent mixture at 300 nm. The concentration of free gossypol in the sample is calculated by referring to calibration curve after multiplying by appropriate dilution factor as shown above:

$$\text{Free gossypol (ppm)} = \frac{100 \times C}{W}$$

Where, C= gossypol concentration (µg/ml) of final solution from standard curve, and W= weight of sample (g).

(C) Estimation of bound gossypol : Estimate bound gossypol by substracting free gossypol from total gossypol.

Bound gossypol (ppm) = Total gossypol (ppm) - Free gossypol (ppm)

•••

Chapter 16

ATOMIC ABSORPTION SPECTROPHOTOMETRY: APPLICATION IN ANIMAL NUTRITION RESEARCH

The potential of atomic absorption spectrometry/spectrophotometry/spectroscopy for determination of metallic elements was first realized by Alan Walsh during 1950. The standard equipment termed as atomic absorption spectrometer/ spectrophotometer (AAS) has now gained a reputation in the field of analytical chemistry for determination of very small concentrations of metallic elements and metalloids. As little as 0.01 ppm of many elements can be determined through this tool. Recently, the Zeeman background correction technique has further enhanced the quality of the results obtained from the flame-less graphite furnace atomizer. Combining the very latest in AA technology with the most powerful computing and software available many manufacturers have developed several designs/models of AAS based on flame or flame-less technique.

Concept

In a simple way we can understand that when a solution containing a metallic salt or compound is aspirated into a flame (acetylene burning in air) the following events occur in rapid succession:
- Evaporation of solvent leaving a solid residue
- Formation of the vapor containing atoms of the metal and remaining in an unexcited state (ground state).
- Some ground-state atoms may be excited by the thermal energy of the

flame to higher energy levels and attain a condition in which they radiate energy.

When the light of the resonance wavelength is passed through a flame containing the atoms in question, then part of the light will be absorbed and the extent of absorption will be proportional to the number of groundstate atoms present in the flame. This is underlying principle of atomic absorption spectrometry/spectrophotometry/spectroscopy. In brief the AAS tells us how much characteristic radiation emitted by the atomic vapour of element produced by dispersion of the atoms in a flame is absorbed and indicates the amount of metal content in the test sample. The source of characteristic radiation is a hollow cathode lamp (HCL). When sample size is limited and higher degree of sensitivity is desired, the flameless atomic absorption spectrometry containing a graphite furnace is used to atomize the sample instead of a flame. The graphite technique is about 20-500 times more sensitive than the flame technique.

Advantages

The major advantages of the spectrometry are:
- Applicability to almost all metals and metalloids
- Excellent specificity
- General freedom from serious inter-element effects
- Good sensitivity for most elements
- Intense absorption leads to determinations at the ppm level
- Modern analytical method
- Simplicity of operation

Limitations

The major limitations of the spectrometry are:
- Accommodates limited concentration range in solution
- Estimates only one element at one time
- Expensive equipment
- Not applicable to non-metals
- Only liquid samples can be analyzed
- Requires a separate light source i.e. hollow cathode lamp (HCL) for each element
- Sensitivity for a few elements is somewhat limited

Manufacturers
Some of the important manufacturers of AAS have been listed below:

- EC, Hyderabad (Electronic Corporation of India Ltd, M 4-5 Stuttee Building, Bank Street, Karol Bagh, New Delhi 11005, Model AAS 4141).
- Hitachi, Japan (Ind Tech Analytical 1290, Sector 29, Noida 201303, Model 1000, 2000, Z 5000).
- Perkin Elmer, USA (Lab India, 606 Vikram Tower, Rajendra Place, New Delhi 110008, Model AAnalyst 100, 300, 700, 800).
- Shimadzu, Japan (Toshbro Pvt Ltd, 602 BDC, Deep Shikha, 8 Rajendra Place, New Delhi 110008, Model AA 6701 6801).
- Unicam, UK (I R Technology Services Pvt Ltd, 204-206 Mohta Chambers, 4 Bhikaji Cama Place, New Delhi 110066, Model SOLAAR 969, 989, 969Z, 989QZ, M5).
- Varian, Australia (Varian India Pvt Ltd, 101-108 1st Floor, Competent House, 7 RBC Nagar Raya, New Delhi-11 0046, Model Varian SpectrAA 220 AAS)

Instrumental Features for a Modern AAS

The research made during the last four decades in AAS instrumentation has brought in several improvements and with the result many commercial models based on a single- or double-beam are available now a days. Since each design is somewhat different with varying requirements of light source, burner flow rate and detector sensitivity, only general outline of a modern AAS bearing the minimum features is detailed below:
- Fully automatic, pc-controlled, double beam optics, multi element, quadline/deuterium background correction (to lower down the elevated absorbance value occurring by molecular absorption or by light scattering), lamp turret capable of holding at least 4 HCL, nebuliser-burner system (to convert the test solution into gaseous atoms), automatic photo-multiplier to work on wave length (180-900 nm), slit (0.2-1.0 nm) selection, monochromator of high resolution (to isolate the resonance line from all non-absorbed lines emitted by the radiation source), detector with read-out system, pc-controlled fuel-gas flow, software for AAS technology.
- HCL having 1000 h of operating life, needs current between 5 and 25 mA and the warming up period between 5 to 30 min.
- Multi-element lamps (have low sensitivity than the single element lamp) are not economical to use, when a single element is being determined and the life of the other element is wasted.
- Optional on-line auto sampler for flame and furnace, diluter, graphite furnace and graphite furnace television option.
- Accessories: air compressor, pc with monitor and printer, continuous

flow vapour system, argon, N_2, N_2O cylinders with regulators
- Fume extraction hood (about 30 cm square) with exhaust fan having ventilation rate of at least 6 cubic meters per minute, located at 10 feet away from the flame).

Preparation of standards and samples

Standard preparation: Ready-made stock solutions for AAS (1000 ppm) are readily available for a wide range of elements and marketed by M/S E-Merck Ltd., Mumbai. Alternatively, the standards may be prepared from metals and metal oxides (Table 1). Working standards should be diluted from standard stock solutions only when needed.

Table 1: Different reagents for preparation of standards of a few elements

Element	Reagent	Weight(g)	Dissolution and dilute to 1 litre	Content (ppm)
Aluminium	Al Metal	1.0	25 ml conc. HCl + 1 ml HNO_3	1000
Calcium	$CaCO_3$	2.497	50 ml 1:4 HNO_3 or 100 ml M-HCl	1000
Cobalt	Co Metal	1.0	50 ml 1:1 HNO_3 or 50 ml 6M-HNO_3	1000
Copper	Cu Metal	1.0	50 ml 1:1 HNO_3 or 50 ml 5M-HNO_3	1000
Iron	Fe Metal	1.0	20ml 1:1 HCl or 20ml 5M-HCl +5ml conc. HNO_3	1000
Magnesium	Mg Metal	1.0	50 ml 1:4 HCl or 50 ml 5M-HCl	1000
Manganese	Mn Metal	1.0	50 ml 1:1 HNO_3 or 50 ml conc. HCl	1000
Potassium	KCl	1.907	50 ml Water	1000
Selenium	Se Metal	1.0	80 ml 1:1 HNO_3 or 15 ml conc. HCl +5 ml conc. HNO_3	1000
Sodium	NaCl	2.542	50 ml Water	1000
Zinc	Zn Metal	1.0	40ml 1:1 HCl or 50 ml 5M-HCl	1000

Sample preparation: The sample to be analyzed can be brought into solution by a number of means
- acid attack (5 ml $HClO_4$ +20 ml HNO_3)
- alkali fusion and subsequent acid attack
- dissolution in solvent

Procedure
- Set up the instrument by burning the flame, lighting the desired HCl, selecting the choice of wavelength, slit width, and lamp current (Table 2) as per the instructions manual of the equipment.
- Prepare the calibration curve from average of each working standard before the analysis of sample.
- The mineral extract in liquid form is sprayed on to the tip of the burner

of specific flame of an AAS. This allows either absorption or emission of rays, which are measured at a specific wave length.
- It is difficult to reduce compounds of As, Sb, Se to the gaseous state, thus the hydride generation method is required which depends on cold vapour technique. Compounds of these elements are converted to their volatile hydrides by the use of sodium borohydride as reducing agent. The hydride then can be dissociated into an atomic vapour by relatively moderate temp. of an argon-hydrogen flame.

Table 2: Detection limits of some common elements by AAS

Element	Symbol	Wave length (nm)	Detection limit (ppm)	Lamp current (mA)	Fuel
Aluminium	Al	309.3	0.3	10	Air-C_2H_2
Calcium	Ca	422.7	0.003	10	Air-C_2H_2
Cobalt	Co	240.7	0.06	7	Air-C_2H_2
Chromium	Cr	357.9	0.02	7	Air-C_2H_2
Copper	Cu	324.8	0.04	4	Air-C_2H_2
Iron	Fe	248.3	0.03	5	Air-C_2H_2
Magnesium	Mg	285.2	0.005	4	Air-C_2H_2
Manganese	Mn	279.5	0.003	5	Air-G_2H_2
Potassium	K	766.5	0.03	5	Air-C_2H_2
Selenium	Se	196.0	1.5	10	Air-C_2H_2
Sodium	Na	589.0	0.002	5	Air-C_2H_2
Zinc	Zn	213.9	0.07	5	Air-C_2H_2

Safety aspects and precautions
- Cylinders must be used and stored in vertical position.
- Ensure that all cylinders are clearly labeled so that there can no doubt about the contents. Always check the gas hoses and regulators for any small leaks in gas supply to prevent explosive hazards causing serious injury and death.
- A flame should never be left unsupervised.
- Application of wrong voltage supply, loose wiring or electrical connections can create fire hazard.
- Fumes, heat and vapours must be extracted from the instrument by exhaust system (exhaust ventilation rate of atleast 6 cubic meters per minute, located at 10 feet away from the flame).
- Always wear safety glasses to protect the eyes from ultraviolet radiation emitted from the flames and lamps.

- Build-up of salt or carbon deposits on a burner should never be allowed to continue unchecked.
- The purity of reagents may determine the accuracy of the analysis and all reagents should therefore be of the highest purity available.
- Standard solutions containing less than 10 ppm of the element should not be stored for more than two days as this will deteriorate due to adsorption of the solute on to the walls of glass vessels.
- Prior to any analysis all reagents and equipment should first be checked for the element of interest by carrying out a blank determination.
- All apparatus for trace analysis should be thoroughly soaked in dilute HNO_3 and rinsed several times with distilled water prior to use.
- Plastic volumetric vessels should be used in preference to glass whenever HCl or strong caustic solutions are to be handled.

Chapter 17

NEAR INFRA RED SPECTROSCOPY : (NIRS) APPLICATION IN ANIMAL NUTRITION RESEARCH

Infra red (IR) spectroscopy is an analytical technique that serves both qualitative and quantitative detection of organic constituents. Near Infra Red spectroscopy (NIRS) is actually a regression technique. Its predictions are based on correlations between spectral information (light absorption) and reference data fed to the spectroscopy. The principle of a NIRS machine is that a feedstuff is illuminated with light of a specific and known frequency (or wavelength) in the near infrared region. The chemical bonds in organic molecules absorb or emit infrared light when their vibrational state changes. In the near IR part of the spectrum, large changes in vibrational state are observed (overtones). In the near IR, 'overtones' are observed (larger than expected energy transitions that occur when molecules get 'over excited') resulting in broad, less well defined peaks. The characteristics of these peaks make quantification difficult as the areas of the peaks are difficult to determine and, typically, indirect (statistical) technique have to be applied to obtain usable data. Water and the C-H bonds absorb strongly in the near IR region, as do the N-H and O-H bonds, but most other have only a weak peak or none at all. The absorption of light by the feedstuff is then measured as the difference between the amount of light emitted by the NIRS machine and the amount of light reflected by the sample. Modern equipment typically uses monochromators, specially constructed mirrors that reflect light in a wavelength-dependent manner, thus allowing exposure of the sample to a single wavelength at a time. This allows samples to be scanned over the entire near IR region (they are also referred to as scanning instruments). However, as the monochromator relies on mechanical positioning of the mirror for its wavelength accuracy, the spectra generated are less reproducible from machine to machine.

Samples those are relatively transparent, such as most gases and liquids, can be assayed easily from the light transmitted (transmittance). For opaque solid samples, however, many problems arise. IR light can only travel through a few microns of opaque material. A few microns, however, can be very difficult to work with, especially when the non-homogeneous nature of most agricultural products is considered. Thus, the major challenge in applying IR spectroscopy to solid samples is sample presentation. For this technique, the sample is put into a cup and illuminated with IR light. This light can have three different fates; it can be reflected off the surface of the sample, it can enter the sample where it may be absorbed if it encounters a bond that matches the light's frequency or, if it does not encounter such a bond, it can bounce back out of the sample. The light bounced back (or reflected) from the sample is captured and its intensity measured.

Win ISI, software for NIRS is powerful but designed to be very user friendly is a product of Infrasoft International, LLC, running under Windows 3.1 , Windows 95, 98, and NT. It is a chemometric package to analyze the transmission and/or reflectance of radiation from solids, semi-liquids, and/or liquids for the agriculture and food industries.

Preliminary Testing of the Equipment : Instrument diagnostics

Instrument diagnostics is to be done on routine basis to check whether the instrument is properly functioning. Diagnostic tests include photometric repeatability, wavelength and instrument response. The instrument should be warmed up for at least one hour (instrument turned on with the main menu "Scan samples" option activated) before making tests. Instrument response is a measure of the absolute reflectance from the ceramic. Wavelength accuracy is measured with didymium (visible) and polystyrene (NIR) inside the instrument. NIR/NIT repeatability is a measure of the deviations in optical (Log 1/R) data at each wavelength and is sometimes called noise. The tests are accomplished by scanning the internal ceramic as a reference, then as a sample, and again as a reference. This sequence is repeated and the two complete scans are subtracted. The statistics calculated is referred to as root mean square (RMS) and root mean square corrected for bias (RMS(C)). The RMS values are multiplied by 10^6 to put the numerical values in a usable range.

General diagnostics limits
Instrument response   Minimum, maximum numbers
Visible maximum   29,500 to 65,00 above or below is unacceptable

NIR maximum	29,500 to 65,00 above or below is unacceptable
Dark average of 3 values	500 to 5,000, above or below is unacceptable
Wavelength accuracy	Recommendation
Visible error	change K and if the ratio of suggested/current is < 0.5000.
NIR error	change K and if the ratio of suggested/current ix < 0.5000.
Photometric repeatability	Limits
Visible repeatability	Upper limit 20.0, above this is unacceptable.
Visible bais	Limit +/- 100.00, more than this is unacceptable.
NIR repeatability	Upper limit 20.0, above this is unacceptable.
NIR bais	Limit +/- 100.00, more than this is unacceptable.

Checkcell analysis

Checkcell analysis is also one of the means of checking the instrument performance and has to be carried out at least once before going for routine analysis of samples. Check files have to be copied intc the sub directory WinISI.

The analysis is made by clicking on the "Routine operation" icon. But before doing the analysis, copy the files from the floppy disk into the sub directory WinISI. Press the "Routine operation" icon and display the "Products" dialog box. Push the "Advanced" button. Then push the "Options" button at the bottom of the "Setup for scanning samples" dialog box. Enter the password "two" and display the "Edit product file information" dialog box. Make sure the "Checkcell equation" is present in the upper window. Go to the options in the lower window and click on "Data collection". The data collection options should be displayed and the filename opposite the "Standardization filename" button. Push the button and enter the WinISI STD filename. If everything is in order, click, on "OK" in the upper right hand corner of the dialog box. Return to the "products" dialog box and make sure the cursor is on the checkcell equation.

Enter the checkcell into the cup stand of the instrument, and Press the "Scan" button at the top of the box. The "Sample confirmation" dialog box will be displayed. Press the "Analysis" button in the lower left-hand corner or press the "Enter" key on the keyboard and the instrument will collect the checkcell scan and display the analysis. The values displayed should not have any change or should be within acceptable limits or else instrument should be allowed for more warm up time or diagnostics test should be carried out.

Calibration of the feed ingredient or test material

There are three basic steps to make a calibration.

Step 1: The analysis is made by clicking on the "Routine operation" icon. "Products" dialog box appears. Push the "Advanced" button and then press the "Options" button at the bottom of the "Setup for scanning samples" dialog box. Enter the password "two" and display the "Edit product file information" dialog box. Make sure the "No equation" is present in the upper window. Go to the options in the lower window and click on "Data collection". The data collection options should be displayed and the filename opposite the "Standardization filename" button. Push the button and enter the WinISI STD filename. If everything is in order, click on "OK" in the upper right hand corner of the dialog box. Return to the, "products" dialog box.

Place the sample into the cup stand of the instrument, and Press the "Scan" button at the top of the box. The "Sample confirmation" dialog box will be displayed. The sample number has to be entered. Press the "Analysis" button in the lower lefthand corner or press the "Enter" key on the keyboard and the instrument will collect the sample scan and display the analysis. Collect the spectra of 50 to 100 samples and store them in NIR file.

The number of sample's cutoff can be set to select whatever number of samples you choose to represent the entire file of spectra. The value of 30 is often used to pick a minimum number of samples from a large file. The neighborhood H will be calculated to describe the average distance between these spectra in options 3.

Step 2: Click on the "View & modify files" icon. Select the MR filename from the file I/O box, select "Reference values" from the menu, and enter the laboratory values. Double check that the sample numbers and reference data have been entered correctly, and exit the program.

Step 3: Click on the "make and use scores" icon and click on "Create score file from spectra file". Enter the CAL filename, push the radio button "Do calculations", make all output files, do not remove outliers, press "Calculate". Review the tables and results and exit the program.

Step 4: Click on "Regression equations". Select "Develop equations with the full spectrum" under "Global equations". Enter the Cal file, enter an equation filename, and press "Calculate". This program automatically exists with the calibration equation stored. Go back to' "Analysis", enter the new equation name in the 'Prod' file and analyze a sample.

Analysis of an unknown sample

Click on the "Routine analysis" icon in the project manager. The first dialog box to appear is the "Products" window. Enter the sub-options for "Equation" and "Instrument setup" to make sure they are appropriate. Decide if output files are needed, press the "Done" button and begin analysis.

Press the "Scan" button. The next display window, "Sample configuration", provides for the entry of the sample number, operator number, and 3 lines of ID for the sample. Below the ID entry lines is the number of samples stored and the remaining space on the computer disk. Press the "analysis" button or press "Enter" to continue. The instrument will begin scanning the sample with messages in the lower left-hand corner. When the analysis is completed, the predicted values will be displayed on the screen. If selected in the equation setup, the Global H, Neighborhood H, and T values will be displayed.

The actual spectrum can be displayed by pressing the 4th icon from the left at the top of the screen, and if the spectrum is to be displayed in hyperspace (3D), press the 5th icon. The current sample will be displayed in blue with a background of green points. If the analysis is acceptable, press the "enter" key on the keyboard or press the first icon and the program will return to the "Select product file entry" window.

Continue collecting spectra and or analyzing samples until finished. When done, click on the "Exit to project manager" button. Pressing the "Enter" key on the keyboard can carry out all scanning operations. When the scan is over, the analysis will be predicted and displayed on the screen. In addition to the predicted values the screen will contain 3 safety test. The global H should be less than 3.0, the neighborhood H should be less than 1.0 and the T value for each constituent analysis should be less than 2.5. If all of these safety tests are passed, the analysis of the sample can be considered accurate.

Remember this analysis program has tremendous flexibility in its operation, the most important part of making analysis easy, user friendly, and error free for the operator. The sample cups are tied directly to the equation. Normal equations as well as databases can be used to analyze samples. All of this can be done in conjunction with discriminate analysis if needed, and or control charts.

Advantages of Near IR Spectroscopy
- Fairly easy to use.
- The rapidity of the measurement - values can be obtained within five minutes after receiving a sample.
- Does not require great skills on the part of the instrument operator
- In situations where an answer is needed quickly, and in such situations a compromise with respect to accuracy is often unavoidable
- For the determination of the moisture, protein and fat in feedstuffs and complete feeds. Presuming that good reference databases exist, IR spectroscopy can be used to predict parameters such as:
- Total or digestible amino acids
- Gross, metabolisable or net energy
- Fat content and composition (including iodine value and free fatty acids)
- Neutral detergent fiber, acid detergent fiber
- Ingredients used in a feed.
- Beta-carotene content.
- Contaminants in products, calculate the digestibility of amino acids in heat treated materials, provided such materials were included in the reference database
- Processing effects (e.g. heat damage from pelleting).
- Composition of meat (protein, fat and moisture)
- Meat quality (color, pH and eating quality)
- Fat quality (rancidity, colour, degree of saturation, fatty acid composition and free fatty acid content)
- Bacterial contamination.
- NIR has shown potentiality to predict the in situ rumen escape protein estimates of compound feeds

Drawbacks of Near IR Spectroscopy

This technique poses several problems; light reflection is strongly affected by the characteristics (e.g. size) of the particle. Light reflection off the surface of particles, however, confounds the measurement and spectral data have to be corrected mathematically for this, thereby introducing an additional error. The second problem is that the depth (several microns for feed samples) penetrated into the sample by the IR light is dependent on the characteristics (e.g. particle size) of the material. These obstacles make accurate quantification more difficult.
- It relies on the data of laboratory analysis and it should be as accurate as possible.
- Large number of samples of each ingredient or feed is required.

- For opaque solid samples, sample presentation / preparation is currently the biggest barrier to IR applications.

In spite of the advantage of NIRR technique there are many disadvantages associated with the same. Infra Red Spectra will vary with different chemical and physical properties of plant parts (leaves, stems and sheaths) and plant species. Each amino acid has a specific IR spectrum and when combined into dipeptide, will have a much different spectrum, which is not the simple sum of the two amino acids. Likewise, different proteins made up of thousands of amino acid combinations will have different spectra. The protein spectra of the sample are modified further by other constituents in the sample. Other factors such as light scatter resulting from differences in particle size and differences in the manner in which the sample was preserved (field cured, oven dried, freeze dried or ensiled). Some other factors, which have not been studied so far, that may affect the spectral properties of the sample, include the soil and environmental conditions under which the plant material was grown. It would be convenient if an instrument could be calibrated once for each nutrient and then never changed. This ultimate objective may be possible for uniform materials such as wheat or corn, but if the instrument is to be used for heterogeneous materials, calibrations need to be made for each product and nutrient to be predicted.

The feed industry has used the technology of near IR spectroscopy for many years with varying degree of success. Many companies have tried but failed, possibly because of false expectations given for the standard of equipment used and the level of expertise dedicated to the task. Several companies, however, have been very successful in applying near IR spectroscopy for resolving issues concerned with feeds; these companies typically employ people who understand the possibilities and limitations of near IR spectroscopy. IR spectroscopy, with its speed, ease of use and versatility, could be about to become one of the most powerful analytical techniques available to the animal production industries. As the method is based on reference, rather absolute, its success will depend upon accurate analysis of the feed samples for a particular parameter, their preservation in the form of sample library to verify the standard graph as and when required and frequent addition of variety samples of a particular ingredient. Moreover, the principle of the instrument / methodology is based on the trueness of all samples of a particular ingredient which may likely to be altered due to incidental or accidental adulteration, which is frequently encountered.

•••

Chapter 18

ESTIMATION OF ANTINUTRITIONAL FACTORS IN FEEDS & FODDERS

Nutritional significance of tannins in feeds and fodders

Tannins are widely distributed in many types of browse plants, tree leaves, forages and feed ingredients. The structure of tannins are not completely well defined but they are polymers of phenolic and aliphatic hydroxy compounds. Although tannins and related polyphenols are considered as protein binders and, protease and cellulolytic inhibitors, they can also exert beneficial effects on rumen fermentation. There are two forms of tannins viz., hydrolysable and condensed. Hydrolysable tannins are considered to have less deleterious effects on protein digestion since these types of tannins might get hydrolysed under acidic gastric condition and release bound proteins. Attempts have been made to utilize this to advantage in protection of proteins from rumen degradation. The condensed tannins are resistant to hydrolytic degradation. The reduction in digestibility due to condensed tannins is not clear whether it is due to specific interference with cellulases or precipitation of proteins.

Certain feed ingredients have been incorporated as a source of tannins, in the diets of ruminants to benefit ruminal fermentation and performance. Inclusion of Bengal gram husk as a source of tannins in the diet of sheep prevented potentially digestible carbohydrate in the rumen, but digested post ruminally (Sreerangaraju *et al.*, 2000). Similarly feeding of tannin containing ingredients such as tamarind seed hulls, Acacia and lotus resulted in higher nitrogen retention, increased body weight gain. The beneficial effects were attributed to the tannin content present (Barry *et al.*, 1986, Pritchard *et al.*, 1992; Bhatta *et al.*, 2000). Tannins present in certain tree leaves and browse plants decrease the rumen fermentation by binding with proteins or decreasing the activity of cellulytics, resulting in less energy extraction from the feeds. Such inhibitory effects have been over come by use of tannin binders. Therefore, tannins can have a beneficial or deleterious effects on ruminal fermentation depending on the concentration and nature of tannins present in different feeds.

Determination of Tannins in Feeds and Forages
(All procedures adapted from Makkar, 1995 and Makkar, 2003)

Preparation of samples

Subjecting feed samples at higher temperatures during processing of feeds can lead to inactivation of phenolics or decrease their extractability in solvents and affects their quantification. Therefore, the following steps have to be followed while processing feed samples for determination of tannins.

1. Dry plant materials at low temperatures, preferably dried in shade, Fans can be used when humidity is high.
2. Samples have to be ground first to 2mm fineness, followed by regrinding of samples using 0.5 mm screen. At any stage of grinding, the temperature should not rise above 40°C.
3. Processed samples should be stored in cool, dark and dry place.

Extraction of Tannins

Use 70% aqueous acetone (v/v) for all assays except protein precipitable phenolics. For protein precipitation assays, 50% aqueous methanol (v/v) should be used since acetone interferes in the process of the complex formation. An ultrasonic water bath should be used for extraction of tannins in these organic solvents as described below.

200 mg of ground feed material is taken in a glass beaker of 25 ml capacity. Ten ml of aqueous acetone (70%) is added and the beaker is suspended to ultrasonic treatment for 20 min (2 x 10 min with 5 min break in between) at room temperature. The contents of the beaker is then transferred to centrifuge tubes and subjected to centrifugation for 10 min at approximately 3,000 g at 4 °C. (An ordinary clinical centrifuge may be used. If refrigerated centrifuge is not available, then the centrifuge tubes with contents can be cooled on ice and then centrifuged). Collect the supernatant and keep it on ice. (Tannins can also be extracted using a shaker water bath, maintained at 30 °C, 130 cycles/min with 4.2 cm amplitude, for 2 h. However, ultrasonic method is preferred).

Determination of Total Phenolics and Tannins Using Folin-Ciocalteu Method (Makker et al., 1993).

Reagents:
1. Folin-Ciocalteu reagent (1N): Dilute commercially available Folin-Ciocalteu reagent (2N) with an equal volume of distilled water. Transfer it to a brown coloured bottle and store it in refrigerator (4 °C). It should be golden colour. Do not use it if turns olive green.
2. Sodium carbonate (20%): Weigh 40 g of sodium carbonate. Dissolve it in about 150 ml of distilled water and make up to 200 ml with distilled water.
3. Insoluble Polyvinyl pyrrolidone (PVPP) (Sigma make, P 6755).
4. Standard Tannic acid solution (0.1 mg/ml): Dissolve 25 mg of Tannic acid (TA, Merck make) in 25 ml distilled water and then dilute 1:10 in distilled water (always use freshly prepared solution).

Table 1 : Preparation of calibration curve

Tube	TA soln.	Distilled water	Folin reagent	Na_2CO_3 solution	Absorbance at 725nm	TA(µg)
Blank	0.00	0.50	0.25	1.25	0.000	0
T1	0.02	0.48	0.25	1.25	0.112	2
T2	0.04	0.46	0.25	1.25	0.218	4
T3	0.06	0.44	0.25	1.25	0.327	6
T4	0.08	0.42	0.25	1.25	0.432	8
T5	0.10	0.40	0.25	1.25	0.538	10

Analysis of Total Phenols

Take suitable aliquots of the tannin-containing extract (initially try 0.02, 0.05 and 0.1 ml) in test tubes, make up the volume to 0.5 ml with distilled water, add 0.25 ml of Folin-Ciocalteu reagent and then 1.25 ml of sodium carbonate solution. Vortex the tubes and read absorbance at 725 nm after 40 min. Calculate the amount of total phenolic content on dry matter basis.

Example: 50 µl tannin-containing extract in the assay mixture gives 0.531 absorption
= 9.896 µg TA equivalent (from the standard curve).
Therefore, 1 ml extract has 9.896 / 0.05 = 197.9 µg TA = 0.198 mg TA. 200 mg of the leaf sample was extracted in 10 ml solvent.
Therefore, 100 mg leaf has 0.198 x 5 = 0.99 mg TA or 100 g leaf has 0.99 TA

If leaf contains 95% dry matter (DM), then TA on DMB = 0.99 / 0.95 = 1.04%

Removal of Tannins from the Tannin Containing Extract

PVPP binds tannins. Weigh 100 mg PVPP in a 100 x 12 mm test tube. Add to it 1.0 ml distilled water and then 1.0 ml of the tannin-containing extract (100 mg PVPP is sufficient to bind 2 mg of total phenols; if total phenolic content of the feed is more than 10% on DMB, dilute the extract appropriately). Vortex it. Keep the tube at 4 °C for 15 min, vortex it again then centrifuge (3,000 g for 10 min) and collect the supernatant. This supernatant has only simple phenolics other than tannins (the tannins would have been precipitated along with the PVPP). Measure the phenolic content of the supernatant as mentioned above (Take at least double the volume (preferable three times) you used for total phenol determination, because you have already diluted the extract two-fold and expect to lose tannin-phenols through binding with PVPP). Express the content of non-tannin phenols on DMB.

Example : 100 µl of the supernatant after PVPP treatment in the assay mixture gives 0.312 absorption.
= 5.75 50 µg TA equivalent (from the standard curve).
Therefore, 1 ml supernatant = 5.75 / 0.1 = 57.54 µg TA = 0.058 mg TA.
10 mg leaf has 0.058 mg TA (since the extract is diluted 2-fold during the test)
Therefore, 100 mg leaf sample has 0.058 x 10 = 0. 58mg TA
Since DM of the feed is 95% = 0.58 / 0.95 = 0.61%
Percentage of tannins as TA equivalent on DMB =
(Total phenolics on DMB — Phenolic content of the supernatant)
Therefore in this case, Tannins = (1.04 — 0.61) = 0.43 % on DMB

Determination of Protein-Precipitable Phenolics (Makkar et al., 1988)
Reagents:
1. Acetate Buffer (pH 4.8 to 4.9, 0.2 M): Pipette 11.4 ml glacial acetic acid to about 800 ml distilled water. Adjust pH of this solution to 4.8 to 4.9 with 4 N sodium hydroxide solution, and bring the final volume to 1 litre. To it add 9.86 g NaCl to make its concentration 0.17 M.
2. Sodium dodecyl sulfate solution (SDS) (1% w/v): Dissolve 1 g SDS in 100 ml of distilled water.
3. SDS-triethanolamine (TEA) (1% SDS (w/v) and 7% (v/v) triethanolamine in distilled water) solution: To 7 ml of triethanolamine add 93 ml distilled water and dissolve 1 g SDS in this solution.

Estimation of Antinutritional Factors

4. Ferric chloride reagent (0.01 M ferric chloride in 0.1 M HCl): For making 0.1 M HCl, dilute 4.2 ml concentrated HCl (37%) to 500 ml with distilled water. Dissolve 0.81 g ferric chloride in 500 ml of 0.1 M HCl. Filter and store the contents in a brown bottle.
5. Glacial acetic acid.
6. BSA solution: Dissolve 100 mg BSA (fraction V) in 100 ml of the buffer.

Formation of the Tannin-Protein Complex

Extract tannins from the plant simple by following the procedure presented in page 40.

To 2 ml of the BSA solution (containing 1 mg BSA/ml acetate buffer), add 50% methanol and increasing levels of the tannin-containing extract to make 3 ml. For example, use 0.90, 0.85, 0.80, 0.75, 0.70, 0.65, 0.60, 0.50 ml of 50% methanol with 0.10, 0.15. 0.20, 0.25, 0.30, 0.35, 0.40, 0.50 ml of the extract (Table 2). This may vary depending on the amount of tannin in the sample. Vortex the contents. Allow the mixture to stand in a refrigerator (4 °C) overnight. Centrifuge at about 3,000 g for about 10 min. Remove the supernatant carefully without disturbing the precipitate. Add 1.5 ml of 1% SDS solution to the precipitate and vortex it to dissolve the precipitate.

Table 2 : An example

Tube	Extract (μml)	Leaf (mg)*	Absorbance at 510nm	TA (mg)**	TA in complex (mg)***
1	100	2	0.121	0.054	0.081
2	150	3	0.167	0.077	0.116
3	200	4	0.234	0.109	0.164
4	250	5	0.292	0.136	0.204
5	300	6	0.341	0.160	0.240
6	350	7	0.422	0.199	0.299
7	400	8	0.472	0.222	0.333
8	500	10	0.591	0.280	0.420

TA, tannic acid (Merck)
- 200 mg leaf is extracted in 10 ml 50% aqueous methanol
- Conversion of absorbance at 510 nm to mg tannic acid by the standard curve
  (see below)
- Obtained by mulptiplying values in the previous column (which correspond to 1 ml of the soluble tannin-protein complex) by 1.5, because the tannin-protein complex is dissolved in 1.5 nil of 1% SDS.

Determination of Tannins (Phenolics) in Tannin-Protein Complex

Take an aliquot (1 ml) of the above dissolved complex. Add 3 ml SDS-triethanolamine solution. Then add a 1-ml portion of the ferric chloride reagent. Record absorbance at 510 nm after 15-30 min. Convert the absorbance to tannic acid equivalent, using a standard curve (Table 3). Multiply the values obtained by 1.5 to obtain the tannins in the complex. Draw a linear regression between tannins precipitated as tannic acid equivalent and mg leaf (in aliquot taken for the assay). The slope of the curve (mg tannic acid precipitated/mg leaf; let it be x) represents the protein-precipitable phenolics in the sample).

Protein precipitable phenolics (x ; mg tannic acid equivalents precipitated/mg leaf DM) for the above example = 0.043/0.953 = 0.045, since DM of the leaves was 95.3%).

Table 3 : Calibration Curve for Phenolic Content

Tube	TA Solution* (ml)	SDS 1% (ml)	SDS TEA (ml)	Ferric chloride (ml)	Absorbance at 510nm	TA (mg)
Blank	0	1.0	3.0	1.0	0.000	0.00
T1	0.1	0.9	3.0	1.0	0.107	0.05
T2	0.2	0.8	3.0	1.0	0.225	0.10
T3	0.3	0.7	3.0	1.0	0.319	0.15
T4	0.4	0.6	3.0	1.0	0.426	0.20
T5	0.5	0.5	3.0	1.0	0.527	0.25

TA, tannic acid (Merck)
* TA solution: 0.5 mg/ml in 1% SDS.

Protein Precipitable Phenolics as Percentage of Total Phenolics

Determination of Total Phenolics in the Original Extract

Take different aliquots (generally 0.05, 0.10, 0.15, 0.20, 0.25, 0.30 ml, but this may vary depending on the amount of phenolics in the sample) of the extract (200 mg in 10 ml of 50% methanol), make up to 1 ml with 1% SDS, and add 3 ml of the SDS-triethanolamine solution and 1 ml of the ferric chloride reagent. Record absorbance at 510 nm as described in Table 4. Convert the absorbance to tannic acid equivalent using the standard curve (Table 3). Draw a linear regression between tannic acid equivalent and mg leaf (in the aliquot taken). The slope of the curve (mg tannic acid equivalent/mg leaf; let it be y) represents total phenolics.

Estimation of Antinutritional Factors

Protein-precipitable phenolics have already been measured as x (Section 2).

The percentage of total phenolics which precipitate protein = (x / y) x 100.

Table 4 : An example

Tube	Extract (µml)	Leaf (mg)	Absorbance at 510nm	TA**
1	50	1	0.145	0.066
2	100	2	0.280	0.131
3	150	3	0.404	0.190
4	200	4	0.532	0.251
5	250	5	0.674	0.319
6	300	6	0.824	0.391

TA, tannic acid (Merck)
* 200 mg leaf is extracted in 10 ml 50% aqeous methanol
** Calculated from the calibration curve below
   Total phenolics (y; mg tannic acid equivalent/mg leaf DM)
   = 0.064 / 0.9535 = 0.067, since DM of the leaves was 95.35%.
   Therefore, protein precipitable phenolics as percentage of total phenolics
   = (x / y) x 100 = (0.045 / 0.067) x 100 = 67.2.

Determination of Condensed Tannins (Proanthocyanidins) (Porter *et al.*, 1986)

Reagents
1. Butanol-HCl reagent (butanol:HCl :: 95:5, v/v), mix 950 ml of n-butanol with 50 ml of concentrated HCl (37%).
2. Ferric reagent (2% ferric ammonium sulphate in 2 N HCl): Make 16.6 ml of concentrated HCl up to 100 ml with distilled water to make 2N HCl. Dissolve 2.0 g ferric ammonium sulphate in this volume of 2N HCl. This reagent should be stored in dark bottle.

Analysis
In a 100 mm x 12 mm glass test tube, pipette 0.50 ml of tannin extract diluted with 70% acetone. The quantity of acetone should be large enough to prevent the absorbance (550 nm) in the assay from exceeding 0.6. It will depend on the quantity of condensed tannins (CT) expected in the sample, and occasionally will need to be determined by trial and error. To the tubes add 3.0 ml of butanol-HCl reagent and 0.1 ml of ferric reagent. Vortex the tubes. Cover the mouth of each tube with a glass marble and put the tubes in a heating block adjusted to 97 to 100 °C (or in a boiling water bath) for 60 min. Cool the tubes and record the absorbance at 550 nm. Subtract a

suitable blank, which is usually the absorbance of the unheated mixture. If the extract has flavon-4-ols, a pink colour develops without heating. If this happens, use one heated blank for each sample, comprising 0.5 ml of the extract, 3 ml of butanol and 0.1 ml of the ferric reagent. Condensed tannins (per cent on DMB) as leucocyanidin equivalent is calculated by the formula;
(A 550 nm x 78.26 x dilution factor*) / (% DM)

This formula assumes that the effective $E^{1\%, 1cm, 550 nm}$ o f leucocyanidin is 460
* The dilution factor is equal to 1, if no 70% acetone was added and the extract was made from 200 mg of the sample in 10 ml solvent. Where 70% acetone is added (for example to prevent the absorbance from exceeding 0.6), the dilution factor is:
0.5 ml / (volume of extract taken)
Example: If the absorbance of a sample (diluted 10 times with acetone, DM 95%) is 0.412, Then the CT content of the sample is
= (0.412 x 78.26 x 10) / (95) = 3.394% on DMB
Determination of extent of interference of tannins in rumen digestion of feedstuffs.
Please refer Section 6.

Determination of Condensed Tannins (Proanthocyanidins) Bound to Fibre Fractions

Condensed tannins in the plant can be categorized as the extractable and bound. The Nutritional significance of condensed tannins bound to fibre fractions (NDF and ADF) is that they might affect fibre digestion (Van Soest *et al.*, 1986). The bound condensed tannins become biologically active due to their release into the medium as a result of microbial action (Makkar *et al.*, 1999). These observations highlight the importance of accurate measurement of bound condensed tannins.

Determination of Total Condensed Tannins in NDF and ADF

Neutral detergent fibre (NDF) and acid detergent fibre (ADF) are prepared according to the procedures of Van Soest et al. (1991), except that the NDF and ADF are dried using a lyophilizer (Makkar and Singh, 1995).
Into a 100 x 12 mm glass test tube weigh 10-60 mg of NDF or ADF. To the tube add 0.5 ml of 70% aqueous acetone followed by 3.0 ml of the butanol-HCl reagent and 0.1 ml of the ferric reagent. Vortex the tubes. Cover the mouth of the tubes with a glass marble and put the tubes in a heating block adjusted to 97 to 100°C for 60 min. Swirl the tubes

gently after about every 15 minutes. Cool the tubes, centrifuge the contents and record the absorbance of the supernatant at 550 nm against a suitable blank (unheated mixture). Condensed tannins (% in NDF or ADF on dry matter basis) as leucocyanidin equivalent is calculated by the formula:

$$\text{Condensed tannin, \% of fibre} = \frac{A_{550nm} \times 782.6 \times 100}{(\text{weight of fibre in mg}) \times (\text{\% dry matter of fibre})}$$

Prevent absorbance (A_{550nm}) from exceeding 0.6. If $A_{550nm} > 0.6$, dilute the extract and record the absorbance. The above formula assumes that the effective $E^{1\%, 1cm, 550nm}$ of leucocyanidin is 460 (Porter et al., 1986).

Determination of Bound Condensed Tannins in NDF and ADF

First remove the extractable tannins by ultrasonication in 70% aqueous acetone followed by centrifugation. Measure the tannins remaining in the residue (bound tannins) using the following procedure, in which the residue is washed twice with aqueous acetone and freeze-dried.

To the residue add about 5 ml of 70% aqueous acetone, vortex and centrifuge (3,000g) for 10 min. Discard the supernatant. Again add about 5 ml of 70% aqueous acetone, vortex, centrifuge and discard the supernatant. Lyophilize (freeze dry) the residue. Weigh 10-60 mg of the residue, measure the condensed tannins in the residue as described for condensed tannins in NDF and ADF.

Determination of Oxalic Acid in Plant Material

Oxalic acid is found in the free state and in the form of salts, both in the vegetable and animal kingdoms. Plants which are rich in oxalates are beet, spinach, rhubarb and sorrel. In contrast, only low levels are found in brassicas, peas, beans, etc. In cattle and sheep there is evidence that the rumen micro-organisms split up the calcium as well as decompose the oxalic acid. In pigs and poultry, diet containing oxalic acid retards growth and reduces calcium retention, although some dissociation of calcium oxalate occurs in the digestive tract.

Method 1 (Abaza *et al.*, 1968)

Principle
The oxalic acid is extracted in HCl and precipitated as calcium oxalate by adding calcium chloride which is then washed and titrated with N/20 $KMnO_4$ in the presence of dilute sulphuric acid at 70°C. One milliliter of N/20 $KMnO_4$ is equivalent to 0.00225 g of oxalate.

Reagents
1. 6 N HCl (Add equal amounts of concentrated HCl and distilled water to prepare 6 N HCl).
2. Methyl red indicator
3. 5% calcium chloride
4. Sulphuric acid in water (1 : 4)
5. $N/20$ $KMnO_4$

Procedure
1. Weigh 2g of sample in a 250ml volumetric flask. Add 190 ml of water and 10 ml of 6 N HCl and digest for 1 h on boiling water. Allow to cool, dilute to make volume and filter the supernatant.
2. Take 50ml of filtrate in a breaker and add 20ml of 6 N HCl. Evaporate the mixture to about half of its volume and filter. Wash the precipitate several times to make the volume about 125 ml.
3. To the filtrate add 3 to 4 drops of methyl red followed by concentrated ammonia (Step 2) till the solution turns faint yellow. Heat to 90°-100°C. Allow to cool and filter to remove the precipitated ferrous impurities, if any.
4. Boil the filtrate, add 10ml of 5% $CaCl_2$ with constant stirring and allow to stand overnight (Step 3).
5. Filter through filter paper (No.41). Wash the precipitate several times with hot water to make it free of Ca ions.

Estimation of Antinutritional Factors

6. Transfer the precipitate to the original breaker by washing with distilled water. Add sulphuric acid solution (1 : 4) till the precipitate is completely dissolved.
7. Warm the contents (70°C) and titrate with N/20 KMnO$_4$ to the near end point. Add the filter paper to the contents, stir it thoroughly and complete the titration.

Calculations

Oxalate (g/100g) = N/20 KMnO$_4$ used (ml) × 0.00225 × $\dfrac{250}{50}$ × $\dfrac{100}{2}$

Method 2 (Cooke and Sansum, 1976)

Principle
The determination in this method is based on quantitative reduction of oxalic acid in colour of a zirconium3, 4-dihydroxyazobenzene-2-carboxylic acid complex.

Reagents
1. 3, 4 dihydroxyazobenene-2-carboxylic acid (DAC) : Dissolve 5.5 g of catechol and 18.5g of aluminium sulphate [Al$_2$(SO$_4$)$_3$ 18 H$_2$O] in 50 ml deionized water and cool it in ice (solution 1). In another container, dissolve 7g of anthranilic acid and 3.5 g of sodium nitrite in 50ml deionized water, and add 7ml HCl (solution 2). Mix solution 2 with solution 1 with stirring at 5°-10°C. Remove the resulting solution from ice and stir (using a magnetic stirrer) throughout the following procedure : After 40 minutes add 50ml of 20% (W/V) sodium acetate solution to precipitate the aluminium salt of DAC. Again after 30 minutes, add 15ml of concentrated HCl and leave for another 30 minutes to decompose the aluminium salt. Filter the cherry red precipitate of DAC through Whatman filter paper (No.50) on a Buchner funnel under suction. Dry the filtrate in a desiccator under vacuum. Purify by fractional crystallization from ethanol in the following manner:
Dissolve the crude DAC product in a minimum volume (25-30ml) of ethanol at 50°C and filter using a Buchner funnel and suction pump. Discard the residue and leave the filtrate to stand at room temperature for about 90 minutes. Refilter and discard the residue. Retain the aerate and evaporate the solvent very slowly from a covered breaker in a desiccator until the product is precipitated. (This may take several days, but complete evaporation must not occur). Filter off the DAC and dry at 60°C. It is stable in the solid state and is stored in a desiccator.

2. DAC solution: Prepare a 10^{-4}M solution by dissolving 0.0258g of freshly dried DAC in 89 ml concentrated HCl, with gentle warming, and dilute it to one litre with deionized water.
3. Zirconium (Zr^{4+}) solution: Prepare a solution containing 5mg Zr^{4+}/litre by dissolving 0.0130g zirconium tetrachloride in 89ml concentrated HCl and diluting it to one litre with deionized water.
   Both these reagents (No.2 and 3) deteriorate after a week, therefore, these must be prepared freshly.
4. Standard solution: Prepare a series of standard oxalic acid solutions containing 0, 2.25, 4.5, 6.75, 9.0, 13.5 and 18.0 µg/ml by diluting 0, 2.5, 5.0, 7.5, 10.0, 15.0 and 20ml of a 10^{-3}M oxalic acid solution (in 1 M HCl) to 100ml with 1M HCl (this solution should be prepared freshly).
   Place 1 ml of each standard solution in 10ml tubes, add 3ml of DAC solution and 2ml of Zr^{4+} solution. The final volume should be 6ml. Allow this to stand for 1 h for full colour development and read absorbence against a blank (1M HCl) at 520nm. Draw a curve of decrease in absorbence vs. oxalic acid concentration.

Procedure

1. Weigh accurately 0.1g dried, ground plant material. Transfer it to a 10ml calibrated glass tube and add 10ml 1.5M HCl to it.
2. Place the tube in a water bath at 90°C. After an hour take it out of the water bath and filter the contents through a Whatman filter paper (No.54) into a 50ml volumetric flask. Wash with 30ml deionized water and make the volume upto the mark.
3. Take an appropriate sample and make a final solution containing 5-12 µg/ml oxalic acid (The final acid concentration of this acid solution should be 1M HCl). Measure the solution against the oxalic acid standard.

Determination of Saponins (Birk *et al.*, 1963)

Reagents
1. Ethyl alcohol (80%)
2. Ethyl ether, L, R., B. D. H.
3. Sodium chloride, L. R., B. D. H.
4. n-butanol, L. R., B. D. H.
5. Sodium chloride solution (5%)
6. Calcium monoxide, L R., B. D. H.
7. Methanol (80%)
8. Dilute HCl
9. Acetone, L. R., B. D. H.

Estimation of Antinutritional Factors

Procedure
1. Suspend 200g finely ground defatted sample in two litres of ethyl alcohol (80%), stir for 12h at 50°-60°C in metabolic shaker and filter.
2. Re-extract the residue with two litres of ethyl alcohol (80%).
3. Recover ethyl alcohol from combined filtrate by distillation in vacuum leaving approximately 400ml residue.
4. Remove the accompanying material and pigments by extracting the concentrated solution with 200ml ethyl ether in lots until the latter is colourless.
5. Add 20g NaCl to the remaining solution and adjust the pH to a range of 4.0 to 5.0 with dilute HCl.
6. Shake the solution with 300ml and 150ml (lots of) n-butanol successively.
7. Wash the combined butanol extracts twice with 50ml of 5% NaCl solution.
8. Dry the washed butanol phase to yield approximately 4g crude material.
9. Suspend 1 g of dried preparation in 100ml of water and then heat at 95°-100°C for 30 minutes.
10. Add lg calcium monoxide to the above saponin extract.
11. Separate the precipitate formed by filtration and again suspend in 50ml of hot methanol (80%). Neutralize with dilute HCl and filter the resulting turbid solution.
12. Concentrate the filtrate to $3/4^{th}$ of its volume and then add 50ml of water.
13. Collect the precipitated saponins by filtration, wash with acetone and dry.

Determination of Trypsin Inhibitors

Principle
The activity of the enzyme trypsin is assayed using casein as substrate. Inhibition of this activity is measured in the extracts (Roy and Rao, 1971).

Reagents
1. 0.1M sodium phosphate buffer, pH 7.5.
2. Casein solution in phosphate buffer (2%).
3. Trypsin (E. Merk) solution (5mg/ml).
4. 0.001M HCl.
5. Trichloro acetic acid solution (5%).

Procedure
1. Take 4g of the finely ground defatted material and treat with 40ml of 0.05M sodium phosphate buffer (pH 7.5) and 40ml of distilled water.
2. Shake the sample suspension for 3h and then centrifuge at 700 g for 30 minutes at 15°C.
3. Dilute the supernatant in such a way that there is an inhibition between 40 and 60 per cent of the control enzyme activity.
4. Prepare incubation mixture consisting of 0.5ml trypsin solution, 2.0 ml of 2 % casein, 1.0 ml of 1.0 M sodium phosphate buffer (pH 7.5), 0.4ml HCl (0.001M) and 0.1ml extract. (In all cases the total volume of the incubation mixture is kept 4ml).
5. Incubate the mixture at 37°C for 20 minutes and then add 6.0ml 5% TCA to stop the reaction.
6. Run corresponding blanks concurrently.

Calculations
One trypsin unit is arbitrarily defined as an increase of 0.01 absorbence unit at 280 nm in 20 minutes for 10ml reaction mixture and the trypsin inhibitory activity as number of trypsin units inhibits (TUI).

Note:
1. *To express the value as specific activities, the total TUI has to be expressed per mg protein. The protein content is generally estimated by Lpwry's method*
2. *The value for trypsin inhibitory activity must have about 40 to 60 per cent inhibition in order to have a reproducible and accurate result.*

Determination of Mimosine in Feed and Faeces

Principle
When a sample containing mimosine is treated with 0.1N HCl, mimosine is extracted into it. The filtrate is treated with $FeCl_3$ solution to form mimosine iron coloured complex. Intensity of colour is measured in spectronic-20 at 535nm to findout the mimosine content (Brewbaker and Kaye, 1981).

Apparatus
Volumetric flask (100ml), boiling batch tube, water bath, funnel with filter paper No.2, pipettes, test tubes, homogenizer, magnetic stirrer, spectronic-20 and wash bottle.

Reagents
1. Hydrochloric acid, A. R.
2. Activated carbon

Estimation of Antinutritional Factors

3. Sodium salt to ethylene diaminetetra-acetic acid (Na$_2$-EDTA. 2 H$_2$O)
4. Ferric chloride (FeCl$_3$, 6 H$_2$O)

Preparation of Solutions

Solution 1 -   0.1 N HCl
Solution 2 -   Suspend 1.5g activated carbon in one litre 0.1N HCl. (Keep in suspension during use with magnetic stirrer).
Solution 3 -   Dissolve 1.0g Na$_3$-EDTA.2H$_2$O in 4 litres of distilled water.
Solution 4 -   Dissolve 4.0g FeCl$_3$ 6H$_2$O in 500ml of 0.1 N HCl.

Calibration Curve

Prepare a calibration curve using solution containing between 0.0025 and 0.025 per cent mimosine in 0.1N HCl.

Dissolve 25mg (0.025g) mimosine in 100ml 0.1N HCl and shake. Take solution and 0.1N HCl in the proportions as given below:

Solution (ml)	1	2	3	4	5	6	7	8	9	10
0.1N HCl (ml)	9	8	7	6	5	4	3	2	1	0
Concentration (%)	0.0025	.0050	0.0075	0.0100	0.0125	0.0150	0.0175	0.0200	.0225	0.0250

Procedure

1. Collect the sample (green leaves or fresh faeces) and dry at or below 40°C until there is no further weight loss.
2. Weigh out 1.0g of the dried sample in 100ml volumetric flask and make the volume with 0.1N HCl (Solution 1).
3. Macerate in homogenizer for 5 to 10 minutes (Bottles can be stored at this stage at room temperature).
4. Take 10ml aliquot of well mixed macerate and add to it 15ml Solution 2.
5. Reflux the contents on water bath for 15 minutes. (Cover the tubes with foil). This achieves 250-fold dilution of the dry matter sample. (Longer boiling is required for very woody samples).
6. Filter through Whatman filter paper No.2
7. Take in a test tube 2.0 ml aliquot of the filtrate and add to it 5.0ml Solution 3 plus 1.0 ml Solution 4. Keep the samples in dark for 15 minutes to achieve full colour development.
8. Keep blank for each sample by taking 2.0ml sample of filtrate with 5.0 ml Solution 3 plus 1.0ml distilled water (in place of Solution 4).
9. Read optical density at 535 nm correcting against a blank for each sample.

Calculations

Mimosine (g/100g) = Concentration against 0. D. from standard curve x 250.

Precaution

Mimosine is highly irritating and, therefore, care should be taken to avoid any contact with skin.

Determination of Nitrate-N

Principle

When nitrates are dissolved in an aqueous solution from dried plant tissue, chlorides and organic matter are eliminated. In alkaline solution, a yellow compound is formed with a phenol sulphonic acid reagent which is measured colorimetrically (Ashton, 1935; Humphries, 1956; Middleton, 1958).

Reagents

1. 0.5% copper sulphate ($CuSO_4$, 5 H_2O) solution.
2. 0.35% silver sulphate (Ag_2SO_4) solution.
3. Sodium dihydrogen phosphate (NaH_2PO_4) reagent : Dissolve 138g of NaH_2PO_4 in 500ml of water. Add strong NaOH solution to bring the pH to 6.5 and make upto one litre.
4. Calcium hydroxide [$Ca(OH)_2$] magnesium carbonate ($MgCO_3$ mixture Triturate one part of $Ca(OH)_2$ and two parts of $MgCO_3$ in a mortar.
5. Phenol-p-sulphonic acid-Leave H_2SO_4 in contact with one drop of mercury overnight to free it from nitric acid. Add 25g phenol (C_6H_5OH) to 225ml H_2SO_4. Heat on steam bath for 2h.
6. 50% ammonium hydroxide (NH_4OH) V/V.
7. Potassium nitrate (KNO_3) solution (standard) — Weigh 0.0505g of KNO_3 accurately and dissolve in 100ml of distilled water. One milliliter of this solution contains 0.07mg N.

Procedure

1. Weigh 0.100g dried sample in a small beaker or flask.
2. Add 9ml of silver sulphate and swirl quickly. Add 1 ml of sodium dihydrogen phosphate reagent immediately and allow it to stand for 2h.
3. Filter and take 1 or 2ml of filtrate into a 15ml centrifuge tube. Add 2 ml of copper sulphate solution and mix. Add water to make 6ml and 0.5g $Ca(OH_2)$-$MgCO_3$ mixture. Mix and allow it to stand for lh and centrifuge.

Estimation of Antinutritional Factors

4. Measure 2ml of phenol sulphonic acid into a boiling tube, directly onto the bottom.
5. Add dropwise 2ml of the above supernatant (Step 3) directly to the reagent, swirling carefully after the addition of each drop.
6. Cool and add cautiously with stirring 25ml of ammonium hydroxide solution.
7. Cool and read the absorbence in a photoelectric colorimeter using a No.42 blue filter setting at zero with water.
8. Prepare a standard curve taking aliquots of standard solution from 1 to 4ml and following the above procedure beginning with the addition of copper sulphate.

Calculations

NO_3-N(g/100g) = Concentration x dilution factor.

Determination of Urea in Feedstuffs

Principle

The sample is suspended in water and filtered. The urea content of the filtrate is estimated after the addition of 4-dimethylaminobenzaldehyde (4-DMAB) by measuring the absorbance at 435nm (Anonymous, 1976).

Apparatus

Shaker and Spectrophotometer with 100 mm cells.

Reagents

1. Activated charcoal.
2. Carrez solution-1-Dissolve 21.9g of zinc acetate dihydrate {$(CH_3COO)_2$ Zn, 2 H_2O} in water. Add 3ml of glacial acetic acid and dilute to 100ml with water.
3. Carrez Solution-2-Dissolve 10.6g of potassium ferrocyanide in 100ml of water.
4. 0.02N hydrochloric acid—Take 20ml of N/10 HCl and dilute to 100ml.
5. Sodium acetate solution-Dissolve 136g of sodium acetate acetate trihydrate (CH_3COO Na. 3 H_2O) in a litre of water.
6. 4-dimethylaminobenzaldehyde solution (4-DMAB): Dissolve 1.6g of 4-DMAB in 100ml of 96% ethanol and add 10ml hydrochloric acid (specific gravity 1.18).
7. Standard urea solution: Dissolve 1.0g of pure grade urea in 100ml of water.

Procedure
1. Weigh approximately 2g of the prepared sample or a suitable amount expected to contain 50 to 500mg of urea and transfer it to a 500ml graduated flask.
2. Add 150ml of 0.02N HCl, shake for 30 minutes, then add 10ml of sodium acetate solution and mix well.
3. Add 1 g of activated charcoal to the flask. Shake well and allow it to stand for 15 minutes.
4. Add 5ml Carrez solution-1 followed by 5ml of Carrez solution-2 with mixing well between additions.
5. Dilute to volume with water and mix well. Filter a portion through a dry filter paper into a clean dry 150ml beaker.
6. Transfer 10ml of the filtrate to a ground glass stoppered test tube. Add 10ml of 4-DMAB solution, mix and allow to stand for 15 minutes.
7. Measure the absorbence of the solution at 435nm against a blank solution prepared from the reagents.

Calibration Curve

Dilute 1, 2, 4, 5 and 10ml of the urea solution (Standard) to 100ml with water. Transfer 10ml of each solution to ground glass stoppered test tubes and add 10ml of 4-DMAB solution to each, mix and proceed as described above. Draw a graph relating absorbence to the amount of urea present.

Calculations

Determine the amount of urea in the sample by reference to the calibration curve. Express results in per cent. To get urea nitrogen, multiply urea content with 0.4665.

Thioglucoside in Rapeseed Meal
The method described will give approximate thioglucoside and isothiocyanates contents in rapeseed meal.

Reagents and Apparatus
1. Barium chloride (5%, solution).
2. Volumetric flask, 600 ml.
3. Steam bath.

Method : To 10 grams meal (defatted by soxhlet extraction) add 250 ml distilled water, hydrolyse at 54°C for one hour and then boil for two hours, keeping volume constant. Filter, retaining filtrate and wash residue three times with 50 ml hot water. Add washings to initial filtrate and make up volume to 600 ml. Precipitate barium sulfate by heating and adding excess barium chloride solution. Leave on a steam bath for a few hours and then filter. Ash in a muffle furnace and then weigh precipitate.

Calculate Approximate Thioglucoside Content as:

$$\text{Per cent thioglucoside} = \frac{(\text{M.Wt. thioglucoside}) \times (\text{Wt. of BaSO}_4)}{(\text{M, Wt. BaSO}_4 \text{ Sample (Wt.)}} \times 100$$

Free Gossypol in Cottonseed Meal

Two procedures are described for the determination of free gossypol, the first for normal meals and the second for meals which have been chemically treated and so contain dianilinogossypol.

Reagents.
1. *Aqueous acetone.* 7 parts acetone, 3 parts distilled water (V/V).
2. *Aqueous acetone-aniline solution.* To 700 ml acetone and 300 ml distilled water, add 0.5 ml redistilled aniline. Prepare solution daily.
3. *Aqueous isopropyl alcohol solution.* 8 parts isopropyl alcohol, 2 parts distilled water (V/V).
4. *Aniline.* Distill reagent grade aniline over a small quantity of zinc dust, discarding the first and last 10 per cent of the distillate. Store refrigerated in a brown glass stoppered bottle. Solution is stable for several months.
5. *Standard gossypol solution.* (a) Dissolve 25 mg of pure gossypol in aniline free acetone and transfer to a 250 ml volumetric flask using 100 ml of acetone. Add 75 ml of distilled water, dilute to volume with acetone and mix.
   (b) *Take 50 ml of solution* (a), add 100 ml pure acetone, 60 ml of distilled water, mix and dilute to 250 ml with pure acetone. Solution (b) contains 0.02 mg gossypol/ml and is stable for 24 hours in darkness.

Apparatus.
1. Mechanical shaker.
2. Spectrophotometer.
3. Conical flasks, 250 ml.
4. Volumetric flasks, 25 and 250 ml.
5. Water bath (boiling).

Method : Grind sample to pass 1 mm sieve taking care not to overheat. Take approximately 1 gram of the sample and add 25 ml of pure acetone. Stir for a few minutes, filter, and divide filtrate into two. To one portion add a pellet of sodium hydroxide and heat in a water bath for few minutes. A deep orange red color in the tube containing sodium hydroxide indicates the presence of dianilinogossypol and procedure (2) should be used. A light yellow extract which does not change color with sodium hydroxide indicates that the cottonseed meal is untreated and procedure (1) should be used.

Procedure 1: Weigh 0.5 to 1 gram of sample, depending on expected gossypol contents, into a conical flask and add glass beads. Pipette into it 50 ml of aqueous acetone solution, stopper the flask and shake for one hour. Filter, discarding the first few ml's of filtrate and then Pipette out duplicate aliquots into 25 ml volumetric flasks. (Take aliquots from 2 to 10 ml, again depending on expected gossypol content.) Dilute one of the aliquots to volume with aqueous isopropyl alcohol (solution A). While to the other aliquot (solution B) add 2 ml redistilled aniline and heat in a boiling water bath for 30 minutes together with a reagent blank- containing 2 ml of aniline and a volume of aqueous acetone solution equal to the sample aliquot. Remove solution B and the blank, add sufficient aqueous isopropyl alcohol to effect homogenous solution and cool to room temperature in a water bath. Dilute to volume with aqueous isopropyl alcohol.

Read samples at 400 nm. Set instrument to zero absorbance with aqueous isopropyl alcohol, and determine absorbance of solution A and reagent blank. If the reagent blank is below 0.022 absorbance proceed as below, otherwise repeat the analysis using freshly distilled aniline. Determine the absorbance of solution B, with the reagent blank set at 0 absorbance. Calculate the corrected absorbance of the sample aliquot: Corrected absorbance: (Absorbance solution B- Absorbance solution A.). Determine the mg free gossypol present in the sample solution using the calibration curve.

Procedure 2: Weigh out 1 gram of sample into a conical flask, add 50 ml aqueous acetone and shake and filter as above. Pipette duplicate aliquots of the filtrate (from 2 to 5 ml depending on expected free gossypol level) into 25 ml volumetric flasks. Dilute one of the aliquots to volume (solution A) with aqueous isopropyl alcohol and leave for at least 30 minutes before reading on the spectrophotometer. Treat the other aliquot (Solution B) as in procedure 1, determine absorbances of solutions (A) and (B) as before and calculate the apparent content of gossypol in both solutions A and B using the calibration curve.

Preparation of Calibration Curve : Pipette duplicate 1, 2, 3, 4, 5, 7, 8 and 10 ml aliquots of the 0.02 mg/ml gossypol standard into 25 ml volumetric flasks. Dilute one set (Solution A) to volume with aqueous isopropyl alcohol and determine absorbances as previously. To other set (Solution B) add 2 ml of redistilled aniline and proceed as previously. Prepare, one reagent blank, using 2 ml aniline and 10 ml of aqueous acetone, heated together with the standards. Determine absorbances as in Procedure I and calculate the corrected optical density for each standard solution.

Corrected absorbance = (absorbance solution B-absorbance solution A). Plot the standard curve, plotting corrected absorbance against gossypol conc. in the 25 ml volume.

Calculate free gossypol per cent in normal meals as:

$$\text{Free gossypol per cent} = \frac{5G}{WV}$$

Where, G = Graph reading
W = Sample weight
V = Aliquot volume used

For chemically treated meals:

$$\text{Free gossypol per cent} = \frac{5(B-A)}{WV}$$

Where, A = mg apparent free gossypol in sample aliquot (A)
B = mg apparent free gossypol in sample aliquot (B)
W = sample weight
V = aliquot volume used.

Determination of Aflatoxins

Aflatoxins are produced by the fungi such as *Aspergillus flavus*, *A.parasiticus*, etc., which grow on certain feed ingredients in the presence of high moisture content (>13%). The toxins exist in several forms, e.g., B_1 B_2, G_1, G_2, M_1 and M_2. Aflatoxin BI is most potent of all toxins. All these toxins have carcinogenic, hepatotoxic, nephrotoxic and immuno-suppressive effect.

Aflatoxins can be determined by the method (Pons et al., 1966, 1972) which involves extraction by chloroform, clean up with lead acetate, defatting and quantitative assay by undimensional thin layer chromatography (TLC) plates. The details of the method are given below:

Apparatus

Conical flasks (500, 250, 100 and 25ml) with stoppers, funnels (100 and 50mm), separating funnels (1000 and 500ml), Lambda pipettes (5, 10, 15 and 25ml), TLC kit and water bath, funnels, cylinder, beakers, etc.

Reagents
1. Acetone
2. Chloroform
3. Methanol
4. Lead acetate 20%
5. Silica gel 'G'
6. Sodium sulphate (anhydrous)
7. Sodium chloride (anhydrous)
8. Standard aflatoxin solution
    a. Stock solution-Four milligrams of aflatoxin B_1/100ml chloroform.
    b. Working solution-Dilute 1ml of stock solution to 10ml with chloroform. Five microlitre of this solution contains 0.02µg of aflatoxin B_1.

Procedure
1. Weigh 50g of finely ground (0.5-1mm size) sample into a glass stoppered conical flask (500ml).
2. Add 75ml of water and 175ml of acetone. Shake for 60 minutes.
3. Filter through Whatman filter paper No.1 in 500ml beaker.
4. Keep it on a boiling water bath to reduce the volume to about 140ml.
5. Cool and add 20ml of 20 % lead acetate and 60ml of water. Mix the contents and filter through double filter paper No.1 into a separating funnel (500ml).
6. Add 25ml of chloroform (first instalment) and shake well. Allow the chloroform to settle.
7. Pass the chloroform layer (bottom layer) through anhydrous sodium sulphate (by taking sodium sulphate on a filter paper) into a conical flask.
8. Repeat steps 6 and 7 by adding another 25ml of chloroform (second instalment).

Estimation of Antinutritional Factors

9. Evaporate the contents of conical flask to dryness (crude extract of aflatoxins).
10. Dissolve the dried aflatoxin in 0.5ml of chloroform.
11. Spot on TLC plate different aliquots (5, 10, 15, 20, 25, 30 and 50µl) of aflatoxin solution.
12. Simultaneously spot different aliquots (5, 10, 15, 20, 25, 30 and 50µl) of working solution on the same plate.
13. Develop the TLC plate in 100 to 150ml chloroform-methanol (95:5) or chloroform-acetaone (90:10) mixture in a TLC tank for 30 to 40 minutes.
14. Dry the plate at room temperature followed by, in hot air oven at 80°C for two minutes.
15. Compare fluorescent intensities of B_1 spots of the sample with those of the standard under ultraviolet light (blue fluorescence) and match the sample portions with that of standard.

Calculations

$$\text{Aflatoxin } B_1 \text{ (µg/kg)} = \frac{V \times Y \times S}{X \times M}$$

Where,
V = Volume in µl of final dilution of sample extract.
Y = Concentration of aflatoxin B_1 standard, µg/ml
S = µl of aflatoxin B_1 standard equal to unknown.
X = µl of sample extract spotted giving fluorescent intensity equal to S, the aflatoxin B_1 standard.
M = Weight of sample (g)

Preparation of the TLC Plate

1. Weigh 50g of silica gel 'G' into a 300ml glass stoppered conical flask.
2. Add 125ml of distilled water and shake for 10 to 15 minutes.
3. Immediately coat five glass plates (20 x 20cm) with 0.5mm thickness of silica gel suspension and let the plates dry at room temperature.
4. Finally, dry in an oven at 110°C for 30 minutes and store in a desiccating cabinet.

Note:

1. After making the final volume, spot the extract as quickly as possible to prevent evaporation.
2. All spots should be of same size and shall not be more than 0.5cm in diameter.
3. Spot B_2 standard solution on different spots of B_1 standard and calculate based on fluorescence of B_2.

4. *The washed and dried plates should be rubbed with a cotton swab of methanol or acetone before the application of silica gel.*
5. *Avoid skin contact as aflatoxins are highly carcinogenic.*

Determination of Uric Acid in Feeds
(AOAC, 1975)

Apparatus
Spectrophotometer, centrifuge and incubator or water bath.

Reagents
1. Sodium borate buffer (0.01M, pH 9.2) — Dissolve 3.8g of $Na_2B_4O_7.10H_2O$ in water and dilute to one litre.
2. Sodium acetate solution, 5% — Dissolve 50g of anhydrous sodium acetate in water and dilute to one litre.
3. Glutathione solution — 10mg/ml in water (Use it within 30 minutes after preparation).
4. Uricase solution — Prepare suspension of 10mg dried uricase in 50ml 0.01M Na-borate buffer (Use it within one hour after preparation).
5. Uric acid standard solution — Dissolve 100mg of uric acid in one litre 5% Na-acetate solution (warm in water bath at 60°-70°C, if necessary). Filter and store in a brown bottle. This solution contains 0.1mg of uric acid/ml. Solution can be stored for a week.
6. 1N HCl.
7. 1N NaOH

Procedure
1. Test for Purity of Reagents
(a) Dilute 5ml of standard uric acid solution to 25ml with 5% Na-acetate solution. Place 5ml each in three test tubes.
(b) Add 5ml of Na-borate buffer to one tube, invert it several times and measure absorbance at 292nm. Absorbance should be > 0.72 which corresponds to 0.072 absorbance unit/µg uric acid/ml final solution. Test standard uric acid solution daily.

2. Test for Efficiency of Uricase Solution
(a) Label remaining two test tubes (step 1a) as No.1 and No.2 and a third test tube as No.3.
(b) Add 5ml of uricase solution to tubes No.1 and No.3. Mix the contents of tube No. 1.
(c) Put a clean rubber stopper on all the three tubes and incubate for two hours at 37°C.

Estimation of Antinutritional Factors

(d) After incubation, mix contents of tubes No.2 and No.3 by repeatedly pouring (six times) from one tube to another and immediately (within 60 seconds) read absorbance of combined solution at 292nm, using solution in tube No.1 as blank. Absorbance should be ≥ 0.648 for ≥ 90 % of theoretical efficiency of uricase. If efficiency is below 90 %, incubate for four hours. If incrased incubation does not increase efficiency to 90 per cent, discard uricase sample.

3. Preparation of Standard Curve

Take 0.0, 2.5, 5.0, 10.0 and 15.0ml of standard solution in five beakers (corresponds to 0.0, 1.0, 2.0, 4.0 and 6.0 µg uric acid/ml in final solution) and follow all steps of feed sample processing except adding ground feed sample.

4. Processing of Feed Sample

a) Take 4g of finely ground sample in a beaker (250ml) and add 25ml of IN HCl and 5ml of glutathione solution. Mix well with glass rod and allow to stand overnight.

b) Add 25ml of 1N NaOH with stirring and adjust pH to 9.0 to 9.3 with IN NaOH or IN HCl.

c) Transfer the contents to 100ml graduated glass tube scraping all material adhering to the walls of the beaker with a glass rod.

d) Rinse beaker with six small portions of 5 % Na-acetate and add in the graduated tube to mark.

e) Shake gently by inverting glass tube several times (every 10 minutes) for one hour (Vigorous shaking tends to produce turbid solution).

f) Transfer the aliquot to 15ml polyethylene tube and centrifuge for 30 minues at 3000 r.p.m.

g) Decant supernatant into small conical flask and pipette 4ml into each of the two test tubes No.1 and No.2.

h) Add 1 ml of Na-borate buffer to each tube and mix by rotating between palms of hands. (Mix solution with Na-borate buffer within 15 minutes to avoid turbidity).

i) Label third tube as No.3. Add 5ml of uricase solution to tubes No.1 and No.3. Mix the contents of tube No.1 by inverting.

j) Stopper all the three tubes with rubber stoppers and incubate for two hours at 37°C.

k) Combine solutions in tubes No.2 and No.3 (as in step 2 d), and read absorbance immediately at 292nm against solution No.1 (blank).

Calculations

Reading of absorbance corresponds to amount of uric acid present in 4ml portions of centrifuged solution.

$$\text{Amount of uric acid in sample} = \text{Amount of uric acid obtained from standard curve} \times \text{dilution factor}$$

Determination of Common Salt (Chlorine as Sodium chloride) in Fish Meal (AOAC, 1975)

Principle
Chlorine is precipitated as silver chloride with a measured quantity of silver nitrate. The silver nitrate remaining after precipitation is titrated with a ammonium thiocyanate using ferric alum as indicator.

Reagents
1. 0.1 N $AgNO_3$ solution — Dissolve $AgNO_3$ slightly more than its equivalent weight (169.87) in halogen-free water and dilute to one litre. Standardize against 0.1 N NaCl containing 5.844 g of pure dry NaCl per litre. Preserve the solution in amber glass bottles away from light.
2. 0.1 N Ammonium thiocyanate (NH_4SCN) solution — Dissolve 7.612 g NH_4SCN (chlorine-free) and dilute to one litre. Standardize against 0.1 N $AgNO_3$. (Take 50 ml of standard $AgNO_3$ solution, add 2 ml of ferric indicator and 5 ml of HNO_3 (1+1) and titrate against thiocyanate solution until solution appears pale rose after vigorous shaking).
3. Ferric indicator — Prepare saturated solution of ferric alum [$FeNH_4(SO_4)_2 \cdot 12 H_2O$] in water.

Procedure
1. Weigh 10 g of fish meal / meat meal in a beaker (250 ml).
2. Add known volume of 0.1 N $AgNO_3$ more than enough just to precipitate all Cl as AgCl.
3. Add 20 ml of HNO_3. Boil gently (usually for 15 min) on hot plate until all solids except AgCO dissolve.
4. Cool, add 50 ml of water and 5 ml of indicator.
5. Titrate with 0.1 N NH_4SCN until solution becomes permanent light brown.
6. Subtract ml of 0.1 N NH_4SCN used from volume (ml) of 0.1 N $AgNO_3$ added and calculate difference as sodium chloride. Each ml of 0.1 N $AgNO_3$ is equal to 0.0058 g NaCl

Calculations

$$\text{NaCl (\%)} = \frac{\text{ml of 0.1 N } AgNO_3 \text{ used} \times 0.0058}{\text{Wt. of sample}} \times 100$$

•••

Chapter 19

METHOD OF CONDUCTING DIGESTION/METBOLISM (BALANCE) TRIAL ON EXPERIMENTAL ANIMALS

The amount of feed or nutrient intake by an animal which is not excreted in the faeces is considered to be digested by the animals. The depiction of digested feed/nutrient as percentage of intake is known as digestibility coefficient. However, this does not represent the true value of digestibility of a feed or nutrient because during the period of recording some part of digested material is returned to the digestive tract after absorption in the body and excreted in the faeces. In addition to this some secretions of the digestive system and debris of epithelial cells are also eliminated in the faeces. These errors are quite large and highly variable for the nitrogenous constituents and minerals in the feeds. Due to these factors the determined digestibility coefficient is known as apparent digestibility coefficient. For the determination of digestion coefficient, only daily intake of feed or nutrients and faecal void values are recorded.

The availability of nitrogenous nutrients and minerals is more accurately determined by their retention (balance) in the body. Therefore, for the determination of the retention of nitrogen and minerals, metabolism trials are conducted. The routes of elimination of these constituents from the body are faeces, urine, expired air, skin secretions and milk (in case of lactating mammalian species). In a conventional balance study the loss of nutrient (s) through skin, being quantitatively little, is ignored. However, in case of some very specific study, collection of skin secretions and materials like shed hair and scurf are collected. For the collection of skin secretion (sweat) a special absorbant suit is used. In all routine balance studies, on male animals quantity of intake and void in faeces and urine are only taken into account.

Procedure For Conducting Digestion Trial

Since there is non-significant difference in the digestion coefficients of feed and nutrients due to the sex, male animals are preferably used for conducting digestion trials.

Duration of Digestion Trial

Duration of digestion trial may be divided into the following two stages:

(A) Pre-Collection Feeding Period

In order to remove the effect of previous feeding and also to adapt the animals On the feed (s) to be evaluated, the animals are fed the test feed for a period of 2-3 weeks. Longer period of pre-collection feeding may be required in some exceptional cases when variation in daily feed intake is large. This may happen in case of non-conventional feeds.

(B) Collection Period

Earlier longer collection period of 10 to 20 days duration was used. After examining the results of different collection periods on the same animals with same feed, a collection period of 6 or 8 days for ruminant and other herbivorous animals and 4 days for simple stomached animals has been found to be quite satisfactory.

Devices Used For Conducting Digestion and Metabolism Trial

Two devices are commonly used for conducting digestion/metabolism trials on experimental animals. A third device is used only for digestion trial and preferably when the animals are under range grazing system.

1. Trial in Stall

A metabolism stall is a special animal house having facilities for offering feed and water to individual animal in such a manner that feed and water of one animal is not used by the neighboring animal. The stall is properly partitioned with strong galvanized iron pipe of about 4 cm diameter. Manger is constructed of cement concrete at a height of about 60 cm from the floor. The inner surface is smooth and inner borders are rounded to facilitate quantitative collection of residue left at the end of feeding period.

The floor of stall is constructed at a height of about 70cm from the ground and space below the floor is kept empty. In other words floor is a roof at a height of 70cm from the ground. A hole of about 3 cm diameter is made at a distance of about 60 cm from the base wall of the manger. This is required for passing the tube of urine collection bag used for the quantitative collection of uncontaminated urine in the recepticle placed beneath the floor. Urine collection is required during the metabolism trial conducted for the determination of balance of nitrogen and minerals, and also for the estimation of gross energy excreted in urine.

2. Trials in Cages

Now-a-days metallic cages fabricated with galvanized iron sheets and stainless steel are mostly used for conducting digestion and metabolism trials. These cages provide adequate space for standing and sitting. The floor of the cage is fabricated to provide a gradual slope from all sides towards central cubical space to facilitate quantitative collection of urine. A detachable feed box or trough is provided in front part of the cage and a window is provided in anterior half of the cage on right side for offering drinking water. The sides are fitted with smooth metallic bars to prevent the escape or falling of the animal. Inner floor space is kept adequate to facilitate reasonably comfortable movements like lying and standing but not turning back.

3. Use of Faeces Collection Bag for Conducting Digestion Trial

A canvass bag with rubber lining and provided with buttoned opening at the level of upper one fourth on the posterior aspect of the bag is used for the quantitative collection of faeces. The size of bag depends on the size of experimental animals and the quantity of faeces voided. Each bag is fitted with strong strapps for harnessing the animals to keep it in position. A, round opening is provided at the top of the bag through which tail is passed out. Another semi-circular smooth cut on the upper part of the bag is provided to fit just beneath the lower border of anus to facilitate the dropping of faeces in the bag.

Feeding and Collection Procedure During Digestion/Metabolism Trial

1. Preparation of Feeds for Herbivorous Animals

The ration of a herbivorous animal may be either a good quality roughage or a diet of concentrate mixture and roughage depending on the requirement of the experiment.

The roughage to be fed is procured and chaffed (about 2cm length) before feeding. Chaffing of roughage is essential for thorough mixing and drawing of representative sample for chemical analysis.

Total concentrate mixture required for feeding during the pre-collection and collection period of trial should preferably be prepared in one lot by mixing all the ingredients thoroughly to ensure uniform composition. Under exceptional conditions the concentrate mixture of same composition using ingredients of the same lot may be prepared in two lots. The feeding of second lot should start at least one week before the start of faeces collection.

2. Fixing of Time For Offering Feed and Collection of Feaces and If Needed Urine

The time of feeding is normally fixed between 8 to 10 a.m. The feed (s) is offered daily at a previously fixed time in the same sequence of animals. This practice starts from the pre-collection period and continues upto the end of the collection period. For a single feed there is no need of sequential offering of feeds but when diet is made of concentrate mixture and roughages, the concentrate mixture is offered first. Animals normally require 30 minutes to 1 hour for eating the concentrate mixture unless the quantity is too large as in the case of lactating cows. Roughage portion of the diet is offered half an hour after eating of the concentrate mixture.

(A) Offering Feed During Collection Period

Required quantity of feed (s) used for feeding during the trial period is brought at the place of trial and thoroughly mixed to ensure uniform composition. Weighed quantity of the feed (s) is offered to the animal at a fixed time. At the same time a small representative sample is taken in a numbered polyethylene bag. The sample of feed is brought to analytical laboratory immediately. Exactly weighed quantity (50g for dry feeds and 100g for green fodders) of feeds (s) is dried in hot air oven at $100+1°C$ at least for 12h to determine dry matter (DM) per cent in the feed. Another sample (10g for dry feeds and 20g for green fodders) is dried in another hot air oven at $60°C+ 1°C$ for the estimation of gross energy.

(B) Collection of Residue

At the end of 24h the feed left in the trough (feed box) is quantitatively collected, weighed and mixed thoroughly. After this sample is drawn and dried for estimation of DM% and gross energy as per procedure described for feed.

(C) Collection and Aliquoting of Faeces

Total faeces voided during 24h after offering feed is collected in a glazed or metallic container and its weight is recorded. This faeces is transferred quantitatively in a large size plastic or enameled tray and mixed thoroughly for drawing representative sample (s).

(Aliquot-A proportion of material (in this case faeces) taken for further quantitative processing is called aliquot).

From the thoroughly mixed faeces 3 aliquotes are drawn after fixing a suitable ratio. The quantity of aliquot may vary from 1/10 to 1/1000 depending on the total quantity of faeces voided daily. In case of large ruminants a single aliquot of 1/1000 size is exactly weighed for DM estimation in hot air oven at 100 + 1°C. Second aliquot of 1/1000 size is exactly weighed in duplicate. One aliquot is collected in a numbered wide mouth and Stoppard glass bottle or plastic container in to which 5ml of 25% sulphuric acid is mixed thoroughly. Another aliquot is dried at 60 ± 1°C for GE estimation.

Dried and wet aliquots of each animal is collected in the same container during the entire collection period of 6 or 8 days. At the end of trial each sample is preserved properly for further analysis in laboratory.

(D) Collection and Aliquoting of Urine

Total urine of the animal on trial is quantitatively collected for 24h after offering the feed in narrow mouth glass or plastic receptacles containing either 10ml toluene or 25% H_2SO_4 at the rate of 5ml per litre of urine voided (approximate quantity of daily urine void is the average of 3 days collection just before the start of collection period). These chemicals are pat in the urine collection receptacles for preventing the loss of volatile nitrogen. The urine is measured with the help of a graduated measuring cylinder. For nitrogen estimation exactly 1/1000 (for large animals) aliquot is transferred in duplicate in numbered kjeldahl flask containing 25ml of conc. H_2SO_4 daily during the collection period of 6 or 8 days. Another 1/2000 aliquot is stored in a numbered narrow mouth Stoppard glass or plastic bottle daily during the same period. This aliquot is used for the estimation of GE and mineral content as per the need of the experiment.

Requirements

For an experiment with 8 animals the following equipment/glassware are required:

1. Metabolic cages (Experiment can also be carried out in metabolic stalls, but for collection of faeces and urine, bags are required) 8
2. Plastic buckets with cover for collection of faeces. 8
3. Glass or plastic bottle (5 litre capacity for sheep and goat and 20 litre capacity for cattle and buffalo) for collection of urine. 8
4. Glass bottles (1 litre capacity) for collections of aliquots of acidified faeces. 8
5. Glass bottles (0.5 litre capacity) for collection of aliquots of urine. 8
6. Trays for estimation of dry matter for proximate analysis in faeces 8, in feeds offered 4, in residues left 8.
7. Trays for drying samples at 60-65°C for gross energy estimation in Feeds offered 4, Residue left 8, Faeces 8.

While initiating the metabolism trial, the following precautions must be taken into consideration:

1. For each diet to be evaluated the number of animals should vary between 5-8 and should be of same species, sex and age. Male animals are usually preferred due to easy collection of faeces and urine separately. A larger number of animals per treatment also helps in elimination of experimental errors and variations from one animal to the other.
2. The animals selected for the metabolism trials should be fed the same diet for 3-4 weeks prior to experimental collection of faeces and urine so that residual effect, if any of the previous diet is removed and the animals are adapted to the new diet.
3. Either various feed ingredients should be thoroughly mixed or their individual intake by the animals should exactly be measured so as to determine the accurate intake of nutrients by the animals.
4. The feed should be offered to the animals at the same time every day and almost equal amounts should be offered daily. If irregular intake by the animals is reported, the metabolism trial should either be delayed or the animal replaced with another healthy animal.
5. After a pre-experimental feeding period of 3-4 weeks, faeces and urine are collected from individual animals for a period of 6 or 8 days after every 24h. For determination of digestibility coefficients of various nutrients, collection of urine is not required. But for estimation of balance of various components like energy, nitrogen, calcium, phosphorus etc., it is essential to measure the quantity of nutrients excreted in urine.

...

Chapter 20

MISCELLANEOUS

Determination of True Protein

Apparatus
Wide mouth stoppered bottle, water bath plus those used for total nitrogen (crude protein) determination.

Reagents
1. Saturated solution of potash alum.
2. Stutzer reagent-Dissolve 40g of $CuSO_4$ in 2 litres of water in a wide mouth stoppered bottle. Add 10ml of glycerine and sufficient quantity of 30% NaOH to make the solution alkaline (Litmus paper). Shake the contents and allow to settle. Discard the supernatant liquid. Collect the precipitate on a filter paper and transfer it to glass mortar with the help of spatula. Add 3ml of glycerine and a little water in the mortar and triturate the precipitate with a glass pastle. Transfer the triturated material to a wide mouth stoppered bottle, add 600ml of water, shake well and filter. Repeat the process till the precipitate (filtrate) is free from alkali and sulphate. Collect the precipitate and add 30ml glycerine. Dilute the emulsion to 320ml with water and preserve in a container.

Procedure
1. Take 2g of finely ground feed sample in a beaker (250ml) and add to it 100ml of boiling water.
2. Shake the contents with a glass rod. Place it in a hot water bath so that major portion of the beaker is submerged in hot water.

3. Keep the beaker in water bath for 30 minutes with constant stirring with glass rod.
4. Take out the breaker from water bath, add 5ml of saturated solution of potash alum, 10ml of Stutzer reagent and stir thoroughly.
5. Allow the contents of beaker to stand for six hours. Filter and wash the precipitate with cold water repeatedly till it becomes free from sulphate.
6. Transfer the precipitate along with filter paper to a Kjeldahl's flask and proceed for nitrogen estimation.

Note: *The difference between total nitrogen and true protein nitrogen gives total non protein nitrogen (NPN).*

Determination of Soluble Carbohydrates in Feeds

Principle
When soluble carbohydrates are heated with anthrone in sulphuric acid a blue green complex is formed, concentration of which is measured spectrophotometrically (Deriaz, 1961).

Reagents
1. Anthrone reagent- Add 760ml of concentrated H_2SO_4 to 330ml of water with stirring and cool. Add 1 g each of thiourea and anthrone and stir until dissolved. Store in refrigerator.
2. Glucose stock solution-Dissolve 400mg of anhydrous D(+) - glucose in water and dilute to 500ml. (Prepare this solution just before use). This solution contains 0.8mg of glucose/ml.
3. Glucose working standard solution-Take 5, 10, 15, 20 and 25ml of glucose stock solution (reagent 2) in 100ml volumetric flask. Dilute to the mark to achieve concentrations 0.04, 0.08, 0.12, 0.16 and 0.20mg/ml, respectively. (Also, prepare this solution just before use).

Procedure
1. Preparation of calibration curve: Pipette 2ml of each glucose working standard solutions into separate test tubes. Add 10ml of anthrone reagent and mix by shaking. Cover the tubes with glass stoppers and place immediately in water bath for 20 minutes. Cool and measure absorbance in a 10mm optical cell at 620nm. Set the instrument at zero with blank.
2. Extraction: Transfer 0.2g of finely ground (1mm mesh sieve) sample to a bottle and add 200ml of water. Put a cap on the bottle and shake (on the shaking machine) for one hour. Filter through Whatman filter paper

No.1 . Reject first few milliliters. Carry out determination of soluble carbohydrates without delay.
3. Pipette 2ml of extract into a separate test tube and proceed as mentioned above (Step 1).
4. Carryout a blank determination, taking 2ml of water in a test tube.

Calculations

Soluble carbohydrates (g/100g) = Concentration (mg) x 50.

•••

Chapter 21

ANALYSIS OF MILK

Sampling of Milk for Analysis

A careful and accurate sampling is of utmost importance for the analysis of milk. It is a fundamental principle of sampling that the quantities withdrawn, must be proportional to the quantities contained in the respective containers and uniform throughout in its composition. Thorough mixing of milk must first be ensured either by stirring or by shaking gently. If milk from an individual animal is to be sampled, the sample should be taken from the middle of vessel containing the whole amount of milk. If the sample bottles have been standing for sometime, resulting in the separation of fat in the cream layer or lumps of fat appear, the bottles may be heated in a water bath upto 40°C to melt the fat before mixing. Milk should not be shaken very violently under any circumstance as it may result in an uneven distribution of fat.

Determination of Milk Fat (Gerber's Method)

Principle
This method involves dissolving of casein and breaking of emulsion of fat in milk by means of sulphuric acid (10:1), centrifugation of the acid solution in the special tube and subsequent reading of the percentage of fat in the graduated neck.

Apparatus
Acido-butyrometer (it is made up of glass and is of about 22ml capacity with graduated stem, calibrated to read upto 8 % of fat. Each small division

on the stem represents 0.1 per cent fat), automatic acid measuring (10ml) apparatus (tilting bottle), pipette (11ml) and centrifuge.

Reagents
1. Sulphuric acid (10:1) - Add 10ml of concentrated H_2SO_4 to 1ml of water (specific grvity 1.820-1.825).
2. Amyl alcohol (it prevents partial charring of fat and sugar by H_2SO_4, keeps the fat clear and renders the separation of fat easier).

Procedure
1. Place the tubes in a stand with opened end upwards.
2. Add 10ml of H_2SO_4 (10:1), 11 ml of milk and 1ml of amyl alcohol into each tube.
3. Cork the tubes tightly. Shake until all traces of curd disappear.
4. Centrifuge the tubes immediately for four minutes at 1100 r.p.m.
5. Remove the tubes from centrifuge. Transfer to water bath at 68°C, immerse it to the top of fat column and leave for 2-3 minutes until column is in equilibrium.
6. Take out the tubes, adjust the stopper to bring the lower end of the fat column against a unit graduation, and read from there to the lowest part of the upper meniscus.

Note : 1. The milk for the estimation of fat should have temperature of about 20°C.
2. If cream has separated, it may be necessary to warm the sample at 38° to –40°C.

Determination of Total Solids

Gravimetric Method

Principle
Total solids mean the residue left after complete evaporation of water from milk. It includes fat, proteins, lactose and mineral matter of milk.

Apparatus
Moisture cup or silica crucible (not less than 5cm in diameter), balance, pipette, oven and desiccator.

Procedure
1. Place moisture cup in the oven for 30 minutes. Cool in a desiccator and weigh.

Analysis of Milk

2. Add 5 ml of milk with a pipette and weigh as quickly as possible so that constant evaporation could be avoided.
3. Place the moisture cup in the oven at 100°C until the weight is constant.
4. Cool in a desiccator and record its weight. Calculate total solids as a percentage of volume of milk.

Note:
1. *Break the skin formed on the surface of milk with a needle from time to time.*
2. *The temperature of the oven should not exceed 100°C otherwise solids will get charred.*
3. *If sour milk is examined by this method, the result is unsually low on account of losses of volatile matter.*

Commercial Method (Richmond's formulae)

$$T.S. = \frac{L.R. \text{ at } 15.5°C}{4} + \frac{6F}{5} + 0.14$$

$$S N F. = \frac{L.R. \text{ at } 15.5°C}{4} + \frac{F}{5} + 0.14$$

Where,
 T.S. = % total solids,
 L.R. = Lactometer reading at 15.5°C,
 S. N. F = % non-fatty solids,
 F = % fat.

Determination of Protein

Pour a known weight of milk (5-10g) into a 500ml Kjeldahl digestion flask, directly on to the bottom. Add 0.7g of mercuric oxide, 15g of powdered potassium sulphate and 25ml of concentrated H_2SO_4. Heat over a low flame till a major portion of water is evaporated. Finally, use a full flame and complete the digestion. Determine nitrogen content according to Kjeldahl method. Multiply the total nitrogen content by the factor 6.38 to obtain protein content of the milk.

Determination of Casein (Hont's Casein Method)

Pour 10.5ml of milk into a 200ml Erlenmeyer flask. Add 75ml of distilled water and 1-1.5ml of 10 % actic acid. Mix the contents by gentle rotation and set aside for 10 minutes. Filter the precipitatd casein upon filter paper

(Whatman No.40). Wash out the absorbed and loosely combined acetic acid by means of cold water. Continue washing of the casein on the filter paper and that adhering to the flask until the washed water reaches a volume of at lest 250ml.

Transfer back the precipitate and the filter paper to the original Erlenmeyer flask. Add 75-80ml of CO_2-free distilled water, 10ml of 0.1 N KOH and a few drops of phenolphthalein. Stopper the flask and shake it vigorously until the casein has been brought into solution. Rinse the stopper with CO_2-free water and titrate the alkaline casein solution at once with 0.1 N HCl till the red colour disappears.

Run a check test parallel with the entire determination. This check titration should be added to the volume of acid used in titration.

Calculations

Subtract the corrected acid reading from the 10ml of alkali used. The difference is the percentage of casein in the milk.

Determination of Ash

Pour 25ml of milk into a previously dried and weighed silica crucible and weigh as quickly as possible. Heat on low flame to evaporate milk to dryness (Skin on the milk should be broken periodically with glass rod). When dry, increase the heat until the contents are ignited with a lighted taper. Transfer the crucible to a muffle furnace and ignite at 600°C for two hours. Cool and record its ash content.

Determination of Lactose (Micro Method)

Lactose is determined on the protein-free filtrate of milk by copper reduction following the method of Folin and Wu (1920) for blood sugar.

Reagents
1. 10 % sodium tungstate solution — Dissolve 10 g of reagent grade carbonate free sodium tungstate in distilled water and dilute it to 100 ml.
2. Alkaline copper solution — Dissolve 4.0 g of pure anhydrous sodium carbonate in about 40 ml of water in a 100 ml volumetric flask. Add 0.75 g of tartaric acid and dissolve. Then add 0.45 g of copper sulphate, mix and make the volume upto the mark. The solution may be filtered, if necessary, through good quality filter paper, the solution can be kept indefinitely.
3. Phosphomolybdic acid solution — Take 35 g of molybdic acid and 5 g of sodium tungState in a beaker. Add 200 ml of 10 % sodium hydroxide

Analysis of Milk

and 200 ml of distilled water. Boil vigorously for 20 to 40 minutes to remove ammonia present in the molybdic acid. Cool it and dilute to 350 ml. Add 125 ml of concentrated phosphoric acid and dilute to 500 ml.

Pour 1ml of milk into a 100ml volumetric flask and add 2ml of 10 % sodium tungstate. Add 2ml of 0.66N H_2SO_4 gradually, mix well and allow to stand for five minutes. Dilute to the mark with water, and filter. Introduce 1ml of filtrate and 1ml of water in a Folin-Wu sugar tube. In another tube, take 2ml of standard lactose solution. Add 2ml of Folin-Wu alkaline copper solution to each tube, heat in boiling water for eight minutes. Cool the contents and add 4ml of acid molybdate reagent to each tube. After one minute add diluted acid molybdate solution (1:4) to the 25ml mark, mix well and read in spectrophotometer at 420nm, setting the instrument at zero against a water blank.

Calculations

$$\text{Lactose (\%)} = \frac{\text{O.D. of unknown}}{\text{O.D. of standard}} \times 0.66 \times \frac{100}{0.01} \times \frac{1}{1000}$$

Standard Solution of Lactose

Dissolve 1g of lactose in 0.2 % benzoic acid and make the volume to 100ml (stock solution). The working solution is prepared by diluting 3ml of the stock solution to 100ml with 0.2 per cent benzoic acid (2ml= 0.6mg lactose).

Note : *For most general purposes, it is sufficient to estimate lactose by difference : Lactose (%) = 100 - (% fat + %protein + % ash).*

Chapter 22

BODY CONDITION SCORING FOR DAIRY CATTLE

Body condition scoring (BCS), although subjective in nature, is the only practical method of evaluation of body energy stores in dairy cows. The method of body condition scoring, originally proposed by Edmonson *et al.* (1987) and recommended by the NRC (2001) is described here. This method uses a 5 point scale, with BCS of 1 being extremely thin and a score of 5 being extremely fat. This system includes a combination of both visual appraisal and manual palpation on 8 separate body locations. Figure 1 shows the suggested BCS chart based on these locations. The assessor can score the cows using this chart with a fair accuracy, without much previous experience of scoring the cows. The scoring method is recommended for HF and Holstein crossbred cows.

Loss of BCS is expected during early lactation when a cow is mobilizing body fat in support of energy needs for lactation. Typical observed changes in BCS range from 0.5 to 1.0 condition score units during the first 60 days postpartum. A 1-unit decrease in BCS for a cow weighing 650 kg at calving (BCS 4) would provide 698 MCal of ME. That amount of ME is sufficient to support 564 kg of 4 per cent fat corrected milk.

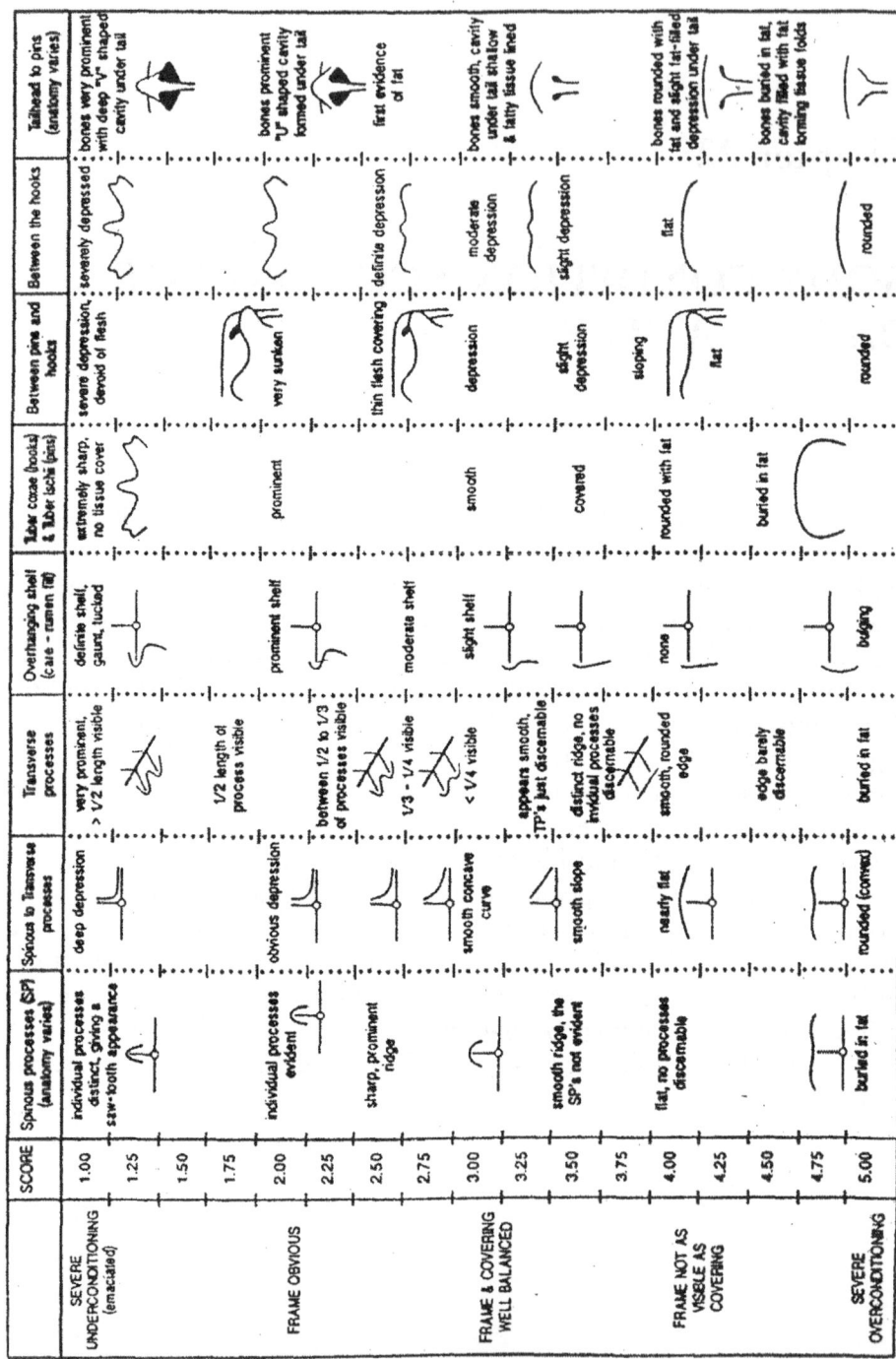

Fig.1 : Body Condition Scoring Chart

Chapter 23

SOME EQUIVALENTS AND FORMULAE FREQUENTLY USED IN RUMINANT FEED EVALUATION

When dealing with the evaluation of the feeds and calculating the requirements of energy and protein for ruminants, it becomes necessary to inter convert values among different systems and units. Since the accuracy of conversions/equivalents and formulae used for calculating the requirements vary with different systems/constants used, the conversion factors and formulae given here can be used only as guidelines for routine purposes in laboratory or farms in feed formulation.

1	ME, MCal/kg to TDN%	Multiply by 31.154 for roughages
		Multiply by 27.635 for concentrates
	TDN% to ME, MCal/kg	Divide by 31.154 for roughages
		Divide by 27.635 for concentrates
2	ME, MJ/kg to TDN%	Divide by .1343 for roughages
		Divide by .1514 for concentrates
	TDN% to ME, MJ/kg	Multiply by .1343 for roughages
		Multiply by .1514 for concentrates
3	ME, MCal/kg to ME, MJ/kg	Multiply by 4.184
	ME, MJ/kg to ME, MCal/kg	Divide by 4.184
4	DE to ME	Multiply by 0.85
	ME to DE	Divide by 0.85
	ME to NE	Multiply by 0.65
	NE to ME	Divide by 0.65
5	Conversion of milk yield to 4% fat corrected milk (4% FCM) yield	(0.4) (kg milk yield) + 15 (kg of fat)

6	Calculation of the daily requirement of energy for lactating dairy cattle (MJ)	Maintenance: 15 + (0.085*BW) Milk yield: 5.2 MJ / kg 4% FCM Body weight gain: 3.6 MJ/100g Body weight loss: 2.8 MJ/100g
7	Calculation of the daily requirement of protein for lactating dairy cows (g)	RDP = 7.8 x ME, MJ UDP = {[(30*milk yield)+75]-[(RDP*.42)]/ .525} Total CP = RDP + UDP
8	Dry matter intake (kg/d) for Growing cattle (45 to 450 kg BW)	$93.5*BW^{0.75}/1000$
9	Calculation of the daily requirement of energy for Sheep and Goat (g, TDN)	For maintenance: $28*BW^{0.75}$ For growth: 2g TDN / g growth
10	Calculation of the daily requirement of protein for Sheep and Goat (g, CP)	For maintenance: $4.15*BW^{0.75}$ For growth: 0.284g / g growth
11	Calculation of ME (MJ/kg) from IVDMD (Tilley & Terry, 1963)	DOMDM = 0.95 (IVDMD%) - 2 ME (MJ/kgDM) = .01554 DOMDM + 0.899

GENERAL INSTRUCTIONS

1. While working with kjeldahl digestion room/bench use fume protecting face mask to avoid inhalation of highly irritating sulphur dioxide fumes.
2. Always add acid to water slowly from the sides of the container near the sink.
3. Never blow the solution left at the tip of the pipette and delivery of the reagent drawn into pipette should be uniform giving appropriate time, varying from 10 to 30 sec. for quantities of 2 to 50 ml.
4. Commercial sulphuric acid should only be used for digestion of samples for nitrogen/protein estimation.
5. Use always glass distilled water while analyzing minerals.
6. During cooling samples in a desiccator, the lid should be displaced to leave a small space, which can be closed after complete cooling.
7. Do not put on fans during decarbonisation of a sample for ashing.
8. Put on the exhaust during decarbonisation and while handling fuming acids and other chemicals.
9. All observations should be recorded at least in duplicate.
10. While opening liquor ammonia bottle, especially during summer season, cool it for some time in a freezer to avoid sudden spurt of ammonia gas accumulated in the bottle.
11. Mouth should be washed quickly with water or weak solution of washing soda during accidental sucking of acids.
12. Acid and alkali spillage on working tables, floors, clothing's should be thoroughly washed with water after suitably neutralizing with either weak alkali in case of acid and weak acid in case of alkali.
13. Consider lower meniscus for clear colourless and upper meniscus for coloured solutions while recording observations with the help of measuring glassware.
14. As a general rule, calibrated glasswares viz., pipettes, burettes, measuring cylinders, volumetric flasks should not be heated or cooled rapidly as it will lead to change in the volume.

15. Distilled water bottles should be kept tightly corked to avoid absorption of atmospheric gases.
16. Always use self prepared reagents and indicators.
17. Always keep decorbonised samples in a closed container like desiccator while carrying to muffle furnace, otherwise being light the material in silica basin may be displaced due to external air movement.
18. Fire extinguishers should be provided in each laboratory.
19. Never pipette strong acids and alkalis with mouth. Always use adopter or rubber bulb pipette.
20. Put on the electronic digital balance at least half an hour before using/weighing.

REFERENCES

Abaza, R.H., Blake, J.T. and Fisher, E.J. 1968. *J. Assoc. Off. Anal. Chem.* 51: 963.

Agarwal, N., Kamra, D.N., Kewalramani, N., Agarwal, D.K., Nath, K. 1991. Hydrolytic enzymes of buffalo rumen: Comparison of cell free rumen fluid, bacterial and protozoal fractions. *Buffalo Journal.* 2, 203-207.

Agarwal, N., Kewalramani, N., Kamra, D.N., Agarwal, D.K.,' Nath, K. 1991. Effect of water extracts of neem (*Azadirachta indicea*) on the activity of hydrolytic enzymes of mixed rumen bacteria from buffalo. *Sci. Food. Agric.* 57, 147-150.

American Oil. Chemists Society, 1972. *Official and Tentative methods*, 3rd edn., Method Ba 7-58.

Anandan, S., G.K. Anil Kumar, J. Ghosh and K.S. Ramchandra, 2005. Effects of different physical and chemical treatments on detoxification of ricin in castor cake. *Anim. Feed Sci. Technol.*, 120: 159-168.

Anonymous, 1976. The Fertilizer and Feeding Stuffs (Amendment) Regulations 1976, No.840. Her Majesty's Stationary Office, London, pp. 26-27.

AOAC, 1975. Official Methods of Analysis. 12th Edn. Association of Analytical Chemists, Washington, D.C.

Ashton, F.L. 1935. *J Soc. Chem. Ind.* 54: 389T-90T.

Aufrere, J.D., Gravion, demarquilly, C., Verite, R., Michalet-Doreau, B and Chapoutot, P., 1991. Predicting in situ degrdadability and feedsproteins in the rumen by two laboratory methods (solubility and enzymatic degradation). *Anim. Feed Sci. Technol.*, 33 : 07-116.

Barker, S. B. and Surnmerson, W. H. 1941. *J Biol. Chem.* 138: 535.

Barnett, J. G. A. and Reid, R. L. 1956. Studies on the production of volatile fatty acids from the grass by rumen liquor in an artificial rumen. Volatile acid production from grass. *J. Agric. Sci.* 48: 315.

Barry, T.N., Manley, T.R and Duncun, S,J., 1986. The role of condensed tannins in the nutritional value of *Lotus pedunculatus* for sheep: site of carbohydrate and protein digestion as influenced by dietary reactive tannin concentration. *Brit. J. Nutr.*, 55 :, 123-137.

Bender, R.A., Janssen, K.A., Resnick, A.D., Blumenberg, M., Foor, F. and Magasanik, B. 1977. Biochemicals parameters of glutamine synthetase from *Klebsiella aerogenes. J. Bact.* 129, 1001-1009.

Bergmeyer, H.U. and Bernt, E. Methods of Enzymatic Analysis, Vol. 2, pp 735 and 760, (Bergmeyer, H.U. ed.), 1974. Academic Press, London.

Beuvink, J.M.W. and Kogut, J., 1993. Modelling gas production kinetics of grass silages incubated with buffered rumen fluid. *J Anim. Sci.*, 7 1 : 1041-1046.

Bhatta, R., Krishnamoorthy, U. and Mohammed, F., 2000, Effect of feeding tamarind (*Tamarindus indica*) seed husk as a source of tannins on dry matter intake, digestibility of nutrients and production performance of crossbred dairy cows in mid lactation. *Anim. Feed Sci. Technol.*, 83 : 67-74.

Birk, Y., Gertler, A. and Khalef, S. 1963. *Biochem. Biophys. Acta* 67: 326-28.

Blümmel, M., 1994. Relationship between kinetics of stover fermentation as described by the Hohenheim *in vitro* gas production test and voluntary feed intake of 54 cereal straws. Ph.D. Dissertation. University of Hohenheim, Stuttgart, Germany.

Botsoglou, N.A., 1991. *J Agric. Food Chem..* 39: 478-482.

Botsoglou, N.A. and Kufidis. D.C. 1990. *J Assoc. Off. Anal. Chem.*, 73 : 447-451.

Brewbaker, J.L. and Kaye, S. 1981. Leucaena Research Report. University of Hawai, Honolulu, Hawai, 96822.

Bums, R.E., 1971. Method of estimation of tannins in grain sorghum. *Agron. J.*, 63 : 511-513.

Chen, X.B., Y.K. Chan, M.F. Franklin, E.R. Orskov and W.J. Shand, 1992. The effect of feed intake and body weight on purine derivatives excretion and microbial protein supply in sheep. *Journal of Anim. Sci.*, 70:1534-42.

Christian, G.D. and Feldman, J.J. (1970). Atomic Absorption Spectroscopy: Applications in Agriculture, Biology and Medicine, Wiley-Interscience, New York.

Conrad, H.R., Weis, W.P., Odwongo, W.O. and Shockey, W.L., 1984. Estimating net energy of lactation from components of cell solubles and cell walls. *J Dairy Sci.*, 67 : 427-436.

Cooke, D.T. and Sansum, L.L. 1976. *J. Sci. Food Agric.* 12: 790.

Day, A.J. and Williamson, G. (2001). Biomarkers for exposure to dietary flavonoids : a review of current evidence for identification of quercetin glycosides in plasma. *British J. Nutr.*, 86 (Suppl.1) : 8105-8110.

De Boever, J.L., Cottyn, B.G., Buyssee, F.X., Wainman, F.W. and Vanacker, J.M., 1986. The use of an enzyamatic technique to predict digestibility, metabolisable and net energy of compound feedstuffs for ruminants. *Anim. Feed Sci. Technol.*, 14 : 203-214.

Deriaz, R.E. 1961. *J. Sci. Food Agric.* 12: 152.

Deshpande, K.Y., U.R. Mehra, P. Singh and A.K. Verma, 2011. Puirne derivatives concentaraion in body fluids as influenced by different energy levels in dairy cows. Indian *J. Anim. Sci.*, 81 (12); 1244-1247.

Dhanoa, M.S., Lopez, S., Dijkstra, J., Davies, D.R., Sanderson, R., Williams, B.A., Sileshi, Z. and France, J., 2000. Estimating the extent of degradation of ruminant feeds from a description of their gas production profiles observed *in vitro*. Comparison of models. *Brit. J.Nutr.*, 83 : 131-142.

References

Edmonson, A. J., Lean, I.J., Weaver, L.D., Farver, T. and Webster, G., 1989. A body condition scoring chart for Holstein dairy cows. *J. Dairy Sci.*, 72 : 68-78.

France, J., Dijkstra, J., Dhanoa, M.S., Lopeaz, S. and Bannink, A., 2000. Estimating the extent of degradation of ruminant feeds from a description of their gas production profiles observed *in vitro*: derivation of models and other mathematical considerations. *Anim. Feed Sci. technol.*, 83 : 171-183.

Giger-Reverdin, S., Jocelyn Aufrere, Saureant, D., Dermaquilly, G. and Vermorel, M., 1994. Prediction of the energy values of compound feeds for ruminants. *Anim. Feed Sci. Technol.*,, 48: 73:98.

Girard, V. and Dupuis, G., 1988. Effect of structural and chemical factors of forages on potentially digestible fibre intake and true digestibility by ruminants. *Can. J. Anim. Sci.*, 68 : 787-700.

Goering, H.K. and Van Soest, P.J., 1097. Forage fibre analyses. *Agriculture Handbook No. 379*, USDA, Washington, DC.

Groot, J.C.J., Cone, J.W., Williams, N.A., Debersaques, F.M.A. and Lantinga, E.A., 1996. Multiphasic analysis of gas production kinetics for *in vitro* fermentation of ruminant feeds. *Anim. Feed Sci. technol.*, 64 : 77-88.

Humphries, E.C. 1956. Mineral components and ash analysis. In: *Modern Methods of Plant Analysis*. Paech, K. and Tracey, M.V. (eds.), Berlin, Springer-Verlag, Vol. 1. pp. 481-83.

I.A.E.A. 1997. Estimation of rumen microbial protein production from purine derivatives in urine. A laboratory manual, IAEA — TECDOC — 945. IAFA, Vienna.

Jamuna, K.V., O.K. Remadevi, T.M. Prabhu and K. Chandrapal Singh, 2012. Nutritional Evaluation of Selected Fodder Aree Leaves by Chemical, *in vitro* and *in situ* studies. *Indian Vet. J.*, Vol. 89, No. 12, December, 2012.

Jeffery, G.H., Bassett, J., Mendham, J. and Denney, R.C. (1989). *Vogel's Text Book of Quantitative Chemical Analysis*, John Wiley & Sons Inc, New York.

Khazaal, K., Boza, J., and Ørskov, E.R., 1994. Assessment of phenolic related antinutritive effects in mediteranean browse: A comparison between the use of the *in vitro* gas production technique with or without insoluble polyvinylpolyrolidone or nylon bag. *Anim. Feed Sci. Technol.*, 49 : 133-150.

Khazaal, K., Dentinho, M.T., Ribeiro, J.M. and Ørskov, E.R., 1993. A comparison of gas production during incubation with rumen contents *in vitro* and nylon bag degradability as predictors of the apparent digestibility *in vivo* and the voluntary intakes of hays. *Anim. Prod.*, 57 : 105-112.

Krishna, G. and Ranghan, S.K. 1980. Laboratory Manual for Nutrition Research, edn. First, Vikas Publishing House (P) Ltd., New Delhi (India), pp. 80 and 83.

Krishnamoorthy, U., Kailas, M.M., and Hegde, B.P., 1998. Prediction of metabolisable energy content in compound feeds and finger millet (*Eleucine coracona*) straw by the summative equations of detergent system and their assessment for application in diet formulation for dairy cattle. *Indian J. Anim. Nutr.* (In Press).

Krishnamoorthy, U., Sniffen, C.J., Stern, M.D. and VanSoest, P.J., 1983. Evaluation of a mathematical model of rumen digestion and an *in vitro* simulation of rumen proteolysis to estimate the rumen undegradable nitrogen content of feedstuffs. *Brit. J. Nutr.*, 50 : 555-568.

Krishnamoorthy, U., Soller, H., Steingass, H. and Menke, K.H., 1991. A comparative study on rumen fermentation of energy supplements *invitro*. *J Anim.Physiol. Anim. Nutr.*, 65 : 28-35.

Krishnamoorthy, U., Soller, H., Steingass, H., and Menke, K.H., 1995. Energy and protein evaluation of tropical feedstuffs for whole tract and ruminal digestion by chemical analysis and rumen inoculum studies *in vitro*. *Anim. Feed Sci. Technol.*, 52 : 177-188.

Licitra, G., Hernandez, T.M. and Van Soest, P.J., 1996. Standardisation of procedures for nitrogen fractions of ruminant feeds. *Anim. Feed Sci. Technol.*, 57 : 347-358.

Licitra, G., Lauria, F., carpino, S., Schadt, I., Sniffen, C.J. and Van Soest., P.J., 1998.Improvement of the *Streptomyces griseus* method of degradable protein in ruminant feeds. *Anim. Feed Sci. Technol.*, 72 : 1-16.

Licitra, G., Van Soest, P.J., Schadt, I., Carpino, S. and Sniffen, C.J., 1998. Influence of the concentration of the protease from *Streptomyces griseus* relative to ruminal protein degradability. *Anim. Feed Sci. Technol.*, 77 : 99-113.

Lowry, O.H., Rosebrough, N.J., Farr, A.L. and Randall, R.J. 1951. Protein measurement with the Folin-phenol reagent. J. Biol. Chem. 193, 262-275.

Makkar, 1995. *Quantification of tannins: A laboratory manual*. Second Edition. International Centre for Agricultural Research in the Dry Areas. Aleppo, Syria.

Makkar, H.P.S., 2003. *Quantification of Tannins in Tree and Shrub Foliage: A Laboratory Manual*. FAO-IAEA, Vienna, Austria. Kluwer Academic Publisher, Netherlands.

Makkar, H.P.S., Blümmel, M. and Becker, K., 1995. *In vitro* effects of and interactions between tannins and saponins and fate of tannins in the rumen. *J. Sci. Food Agric.*, 69 : 481-493.

Makkar, H.P.S., Blümmel, M. and Becker, K., 1995. Formation of complexes between polyvinyl pyrrolidones and polyethylene glycols with tannins and their implications in gas production and true digestibility in vitro techniques. *Brit. J.Nutr.*, 73 : 897 - 913.

Makkar, H.P.S., Blümmel, M., Borowy, N.K. and Becker, K., 1993. Gravimetric determination of tanninsand their correlations with chemical and protein precipitation methods. *J. Sci. Food. Agric.*, 61 : 161-165.

Makkar, H.P.S., Dawra, R.K and Singh, B., 1988. Determination of both tannin and protein in a tannin-protein complex. *J. Agric. Food Chem.*, 36 : 523-525.

Mansell,R.E. and Enmel,H.W. 1965. *Atomic Absorption News letter*, 4: 365.

Marten, G.C. and Barnes,R.F., 1979. Prediction of energy digestibility of forages with *in vitro* rumen fermentation and fungal enzyme systems. In: Pigden,

References

W.J., Balch, C.C. and Graham, M. (Eds). Standardisation od Analytical Methodology for feeds. IDRC, Ottawa, Canada.

Meers, J.L., Tempest, D.W. and Brown, C.M. 1970. Glutamine (amide): 2-oxoglutarate amino transferase oxido-reductase (NADP) an enzyme involved in the synthesis of glutamate by some bacteria. *J. Gen. Microbiol.* 64: 187-194.

Menke, K.H. and Steingass, H., 1988. Estimation of the energetic fed value obtained from chemical analysis and *in vitro* gas production using rumen fluid. *Anim.Res.Dev.*, 28 : 7-55.

Menke, K.H., Raab, L., Salewski, A., Steingass, H., Fritz, D. and Schneider, W., 1979. The estimation of digestibility and metabolisable energy content of ruminant feedstuffs from the gas production when they are incubated with rumen liquor *in vitro. J. Agric.Sci.*, 93 : 217-222.

Merken, H.M. and Beecher, G.R. (2000). Measurement of food flavonoids by HPLC-a review. *J Agric. Food Chern.*, 48: 577-599.

Middleton, K.R. 1958. *J Appl. Chem.* 8: 99-08.

Miller, G.L. 1959. Use of dinitrosalicylic acid reagent for determination of reducing sugar. *Anal. Chem.* 31: 426-428.

Morgan, M.E. 1964. Atomic Absorption News letter, Perkin. Elmer Corporation, Norwalk, Connecticut.

Mota, M., J., Balacells, N.H. Ozdemir Baber, S. Boulklepe and A. Belengner, 2008. Modeling purine derivatives excretion in dairy goats: endogenous excretion and the relationship between duodenal input and urinary output. *Animal* 2(1):44-51.

Nataraja, M.B., Krishnamoorthy, U. and Krishnappa, P., 1998. Assessment of rumen *in vitro* incubation (Gas production) technique and chemical analysis by detergent system to predict metabolisable energy content in mixed diets of lactating cows. *Anim. Feed Sci. technol.*, 74 : 169-177.

National Research Council (NRC), 2001. Nutrient Requirements of Dairy Cattle, 7th Revised Edition, National Academy Press, Washington, DC, pp 23-25.

Nocek, J.E., 1988. In situ and other methods to estimate ruminal protein and energy digestivility: a review. *J. Dairy Sci.*, 71 : 2051-2069.

Ørskov, E.R. and McDonald, I., 1979. The estimation of protein degradability in the rumen from incubation measurements weighted according to the rate of passage. *J Agric. Sci. Camb.*, 92 : 499-503.

Pell, A.N. and Schofield, P. 1993. Computerised monitoring of gas production to measure forage digestion *in vitro. J. Dairy Sci.*, 76 : 1063-1073.

Pichard, G.R. and Van Soest, P.J., 1977. Protein solubility in ruminant feeds. Proc. Cornell Nutr.Conf. for feed manufacturers. Pp 91-95.

Pichard. D.A., Martin, P.R. and O'Rovike, P.K., 1992. The role of condensed tannins in the nutritional value of Mulgs (*Acacia aneura*) for sheep. *Aus. J. Agric. Res.*, 43 : 1739-1746.

Pickett, E.E. and Koirtyohann, S.R. 1968. *Spectrochimica Acta*, 23B:235.

Pickett, E.E. and Koirtyohann, S.R. 1969. *Analyt. Chem.*, 14:28A.

Pons, W.A. Jr., Cucullu, A.F., Lee, L.S., Franz, A.O. and Goldblatt, L.A. 1966. *J. Assoc. Off Anal. Chem.* 49: 554-62.

Pons, W.A., Cucullu, A.F. and Franz, A.O. 1972. *J. Assoc. Off. Anal. Chem.* 55: 768-74.

Porter, L.J., Hrstich, L.N. and Chan, B.G., 1986. The conversion of procyanidins and prodelphinidins to cyanidin and delphinidin. *Phytochemistry*, 25 : 223-230.

Prabhu, T.M., C.Devakumar, V.R.B. Sastry and D.K. Agarwal. 2002. Identification of Karanjin using HPLC in raw and detoxified karanj seed cake. *Asian-Aust. J. Anim.Sci.*, 15(3): 416-420.

Prabhu, T.M, Farooq Mohammed, U.Krishnamoorthy and K.Chandrapal Singh. 1998. *In vitro* protease technique as an alternative for in situ method of estimating degradable protein. *Indian J. Anim. Sci.* 68(02):1287-1289.

Prabhu, T.M, Farooq Mohammed, U.Krishnamoorthy and K.Chandrapal Singh. 1996. Comparitive study of rumen degradability of protein by *in situ* and *in vitro* (protease) techniques. *Indian J. Anim.Nutr.* 34 (4):190-196.

Prabhu.T.M,V.R.B.Sastry,FarooqMohammedandK.ChandrapalSingh.1999.*In situ* and *In vitro* methods for estimation of rumen degradable protein and undegradable dietary protein. A Review. *Indian J.Dairy.Biosci.*10: 1-8.

Price, W.J. (1974). *Analytical Atomic Absorption Spectrometry*, Heyden & Sons Ltd., London.

Raab, L., Cafantaris, B.,Jilg, T. and Manke, K.H., 1983. Rumen protein degradation and biosynthesis. 1. A new method of determination of protein degradation in rumen fluid *in vitro*. *Brit. J. Nutr.*, 50 : 560-582.

Ramagaokar,J.S., A.K. Verma, P. Singh and U.R. Mehra, 2008. Effect of dietary protein levels on urinary excretion and plasma concentration of purine derivatives in crossbred bulls. *Anim. Nutr. and Feed Technol.*, 8:25-34.

Reitman, S. and Frankel, S. 1957. Determination of serum glutamic oxaloacetic transaminase and pyruvic transaminase by colorimetric method. *Amer. J. Clin. Pathol.* 28: 56.

Renuka, B.C., K.Chandrapal Singh and T.M.Prabhu.2003. Efficiency of internal markers for predicting nutrient digestibility in dairy cows. *Indian. J. Anim. Nutr. Feed Technol.* 3(2): 159-164.

Reynolds, R.J., Aldous, K. and Thompson, K.C. (1970). Atomic Absorption Spectroscopy, Griffin, London.

Roy, D.N. and Rao, P.S. 1971. *J. Agric. Food Chem.* 19: 257-59.

Sastry, V.R.B., D.N. Kamra and N.N. Pathak. 1999. Laboratory manual of Animal Nutrition. IVRI, Izatnagar, UP, India.

Shewale, J.G. and Sadana, J.C. 1978. Cellulase and β-glucosidase by a basidomycete species. *Can. J. Microbiol.* 24: 1204-1216.

Singh, M.K. Sharma, N. Datta, P. Singh, A.K. Verma and U.R. Mehra, 2007. Estimation of rumen microbial protein supply using purine derivatives excretion in cossbred calves fed at different levels of feed intake. *Asian-Austral. J. Anim. Sci.*, 20(10): 1567-74.

Smith, R.H. (1959). The development and function of the rumen in milk fed calves. *J. Agric. Sci.* 52: 72-78.

Smith, R.H. (1970). Nucleic acid metabolism in the ruminant. *British J. Nutr.* 24: 545-56.

References

Sreerangaraju, G., Krishnamoorthy, U. and Kailas, M.M., 2000. Evaluation of Bengal gram (*Cicer arietinum*) husk as a source of tannin and its interference in rumen and post rumen nutrient digestion in sheep. *Anim Feed Sci. Technol.*, 85 : 131-138.

Susmel, P., Stenfanin, E. Plazzota, M. Spanghero and C.R. Mills. 1994. The effect of energy and protein intake on the excretion of purine derivatives. *Journal Agric. Sci. Cambri.*, 123: 257-65.

Theodorou, M.K., Williams, B.A., Dhanoa, M.S., McAllan, A.B. and France, J., 1994. A simple gas production method using a pressure transducer to determine the fermentation kinetics of ruminant feeds. *Anim. Feed Sci. Technol.*, 48 : 185-198.

Tilley, J.M.A. and Terry, R.A., 1963. A two-stage technique for *in vitro* digestion of forage crops. *J Brit. Grassland Soc.*, 18 : 104-111.

Van Soest, P.J., 1971. Estimation of nutritive value from laboratory analysis. Proc. Cornell Nutr.Conf. for the feed manufacturers. P 106-117.

Van Soest, P.J., 1982. Nutritional Ecology of the Ruminants. 1st Ed., O and B Books, Corvallis, Oregon, USA.

Van Soest, P.J., 1994. Nutritional Ecology of the Ruminants. 2nd Ed. Cornell University Press, Ithaca, New York, USA.

Wilson, K. and Walker, J. (1994). Principles and techniques of practical Biochemistry. pp 462-529.

Wolf, P.L., Williams, D. 1973. Practical clinical enzymology: Techniques and interpretations. Wiley-Interscience Publication, New York.

Zettner A., Sylva, L.C. and Capacho Delgado, L. 1966. *Am.J.Clin.Path.*, 45:533.

Printed and bound by CPI Group (UK) Ltd, Croydon, CR0 4YY
22/04/2026

14866396-0002